Self-Assessment Colour Review of

Small Animal Abdominal and Metabolic Disorders

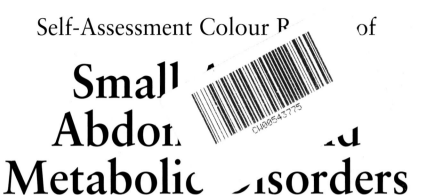

Bryn Tennant
BVSc, PhD, CertVR, MRCVS
Capital Diagnostics
SAC Veterinary Science Division
Penicuik, Midlothian, UK

Manson Publishing/The Veterinary Press

Acknowledgements

Illustrations **67** and **74** are reproduced with permission of Dr F. J. McEvoy; **88a** and **b** with permission of Mr M. E. Herrtage; and **99** with permission of Dr K. Monce.

For full details of all Manson Publishing titles, please write to:
Manson Publishing Ltd, 73 Corringham Road, London NW11 7DL, UK.

Project management: Paul Bennett
Text editing: Peter Beynon
Design and layout: Patrick Daly and Lara Last
Colour reproduction: Tenon & Polert Colour Scanning Ltd, Hong Kong
Printed by: Grafos SA, Barcelona, Spain

Preface

Veterinary medicine continues to evolve and progress as concepts change, new disorders are recognized and novel diagnostic approaches are reported. This book brings together a wide variety of cases and clinical situations which relate to disorders of the abdominal cavity in a question and answer format. These cases are presented in different ways and relate to the highly individual approach to cases by each of the wide variety of specialist authors who have contributed to the text. The book should be useful to all veterinary surgeons and students and provides a rich mix of material ranging from relatively simple cases to complex and controversial subjects. It is hoped that the text will not only serve to test the ability of the reader but also be informative.

The cases primarily draw on diseases affecting organs of the abdominal cavity, although non-abdominal disorders primarily relating to endocrine problems, and occasional muscular, neurological and dermatological disorders, are also included. The different subject areas are randomly mixed throughout the book. The Broad Classification of Cases (below) and the Index (page 191) can be used to find specific areas of interest. Normal biochemical and haematological values are listed in the Appendix (page 189). The results within the body of the text use SI units, but old units are included in the Appendix along with conversion factors. The abbreviations used within the text are listed on the inside of the front cover.

Broad Classification of Cases

Body cavities   19, 36, 45, 46, 74, 148, 165, 187
Cardiovascular 33, 45
Endocrine 5, 14, 23, 30, 41, 47, 52, 53, 93, 100, 107, 121, 123, 140, 142, 145, 149, 157, 163
Haematology 2, 8, 31, 69, 73, 95, 102, 110, 112, 124, 132, 191
Infectious disease 9, 16, 18, 24, 38, 39, 40, 44, 48, 57, 62, 63, 70, 81, 82, 83, 90, 98, 99, 103, 122, 124, 147, 158, 161, 170, 176, 184, 188
Intestine 6, 13, 29, 54, 55, 61, 62, 76, 81, 88, 94, 101, 116, 119, 120, 127, 131, 141, 147, 153, 161, 162, 166, 175, 186, 189, 195
Kidney 1, 7, 27, 32, 49, 58, 72, 79, 80, 84, 87, 96, 104, 108, 111, 117, 122, 137, 144, 150, 155, 173, 182, 193, 196
Liver 20, 22, 26, 37, 46, 56, 64, 65, 67, 71, 74, 77, 89, 92, 130, 146, 151, 154,
156, 160, 168, 174, 177, 178, 187, 193
Lower urinary tract 4, 10, 32, 42, 75, 106, 113, 118, 126, 129, 133, 135, 138, 143
Neoplasia 1, 8, 21, 25, 54, 59, 85, 92, 133, 146, 164, 172, 173, 180, 183
Neurology 39, 70, 171, 177
Nutrition 13, 15, 34, 64, 71, 101, 134, 186, 190, 195
Oesophagus 34, 68, 128, 159
Ophthalmology 33, 142, 167
Orthopaedic 85, 98, 182
Pancreas 25, 127, 152, 174
Prostate 35, 97, 106, 139
Reproduction 11, 17, 28, 50, 51, 60, 66, 78, 86, 105, 109, 114, 176, 180
Respiratory 6, 63, 170
Skin 37, 186
Stomach 3, 12, 15, 25, 68, 72, 91, 99, 103, 115, 119, 125, 136, 164, 181, 183, 185, 192
Toxins 102, 104

3

Contributors

Diane Addie, BVMS PhD MRCVS
University of Glasgow Veterinary School
Department of Veterinary Pathology
Bearsden, Glasgow G61 1QH, UK

Joe Bartges, DVM
University of Georgia
College of Veterinary Medicine
Department of Small Animal Medicine
and Surgery
Athens, GA 3060L, USA

Gary England, BVetMed PhD DVR
CertVA DVRep DipACT FRCVS
Royal Veterinary College
Department of Small Animal Medicine
and Surgery
Hatfield, Hertfordshire AL9 7TA, UK

Sue Gregory, BVetMed PhD DVR DSAS
MRCVS
Royal Veterinary College
Department of Small Animal Medicine
and Surgery
Hatfield, Hertfordshire AL9 7T, UK

Ed Hall, MA VetMB PhD MRCVS
University of Bristol
Department of Clinical Veterinary
Science
Langford, Bristol BS18 7DU, UK

Karyl Hurley, DVM
Royal Veterinary College
Department of Small Animal Medicine
and Surgery
Hatfield, Hertfordshire AL9 7TA, UK

Carmel Mooney, MVB MPhil MRCVS
Department of Small Animal Clinical
Studies, Faculty of Veterinary Medicine
University College Dublin
Ballsbridge, Dublin 4, Ireland

Carolien Rutgers, DVM MS DipACVIM
DSAM MRCVS
Royal Veterinary College
Department of Small Animal Medicine
and Surgery
Hatfield, Hertfordshire AL9 7TA, UK

Andrew Sparkes, BVetMed PhD MRCVS
University of Bristol
Department of Clinical Veterinary
Science
Langford, Bristol BS18 7DU, UK

Bryn Tennant, BVSc PhD CertVR
MRCVS
Capital Diagnostics
SAC Veterinary Science Divison
Penicuik, Midlothian EH26 0QE, UK

Andrew Torrance, MA VetMB PhD
DipACVIM MRCVS
Bloxham Laboratories
Teignmouth, Devon TQ14 8AH, UK

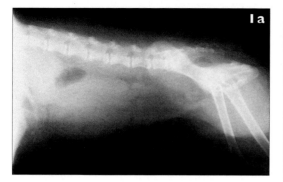

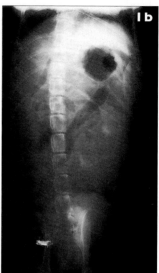

1 Lateral survey radiograph (**1a**) and ventrodorsal abdominal radiograph (**1b**) taken 20 minutes after intravenous administration of contrast media to a nine-year-old, neutered female Lhasa Apso with a two-week history of haematuria. Abdominal palpation revealed a mid-abdominal mass.
i. What is your diagnosis?
ii. What is the commonest type of renal neoplasm in dogs?
iii. What is the commonest type of renal neoplasm in cats?

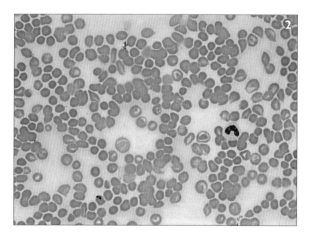

2 Examine the RBC morphology and arrangement shown (**2**).
i. Comment on the findings in the film.
ii. Would these microscopic findings be evident grossly in the sample?
iii. What is the significance of these findings?
iv. Would you elect to perform a Coombs test in this case?

1 i. Abdominal mass located in the area of one of the kidneys. The contrast material has outlined the mass, confirming it as a kidney. Intravenous pyelography increases the accuracy of demonstrating suspicious abdominal masses as a kidney. A blush in one area of the kidney may be seen due to neovascularization associated with the tumour. On occasions there may be little or no uptake of contrast material. The mass was removed surgically (**1c**).

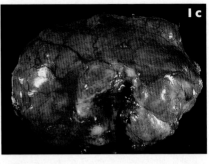

ii. Over 85% of canine kidney tumours are epithelial and 90% are malignant. Two thirds of renal neoplasms are carcinomas. Other tumours include transitional cell carcinoma, adenoma, papilloma, fibroma, lymphoma, sarcoma and nephroblastoma.

iii. In cats the commonest renal neoplasm is lymphosarcoma which usually affects both kidneys. Approximately 50% of cats with renal lymphoma test positive for FeLV and approximately 40% of cats with renal lymphoma also have CNS involvement. Other cancers affecting feline kidneys include carcinoma and nephroblastoma.

2 i. The RBCs show anisocytosis and polychromasia. The clumped pattern of the RBCs is due to agglutination. Microscopically this can usually be differentiated from rouleaux formation which appears as stacked arrays of RBCs rather than clumps.

ii. This is microscopic agglutination; the clumps are not large enough to be visible grossly. When clumps of RBCs can be seen grossly in the sample they must be differentiated from rouleaux formation by mixing one drop of blood with one drop of normal saline on a slide. The rouleaux will disperse, while agglutination will persist.

iii. The microscopic agglutination implies that RBCs are bound together by antibodies or complement and suggests an immunological disease process. This sample shows evidence of regeneration and it is fair to assume that this is a case of autoimmune haemolytic anaemia (AIHA).

iv. Where the haematological profile findings are consistent with AIHA and microagglutination is present, demonstrating the presence of antibody or complement bound to RBCs using a Coombs test yields no further diagnostic information; the diagnosis of AIHA has already been made. Coombs tests quite frequently give anomalous or unreliable results when performed on samples already containing agglutinated RBCs.

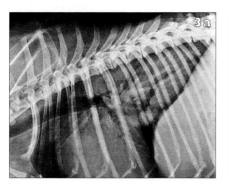 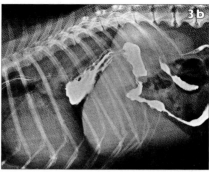

3 This radiograph (3a) is of a four-year-old, entire male Yorkshire Terrier who had a history of intermittent, passive regurgitation of food and water for several years. Thoracic radiographs were taken and subsequent contrast radiography was performed (3b).
i. Describe your radiographic findings, and state your diagnosis.
ii. What therapy do you recommend?

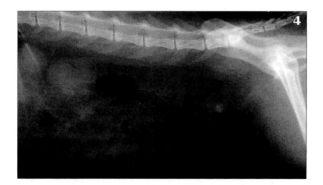

4 A seven-year-old, neutered female cat was presented with a history of intermittent haematuria over the last six months which responded to treatment with antibiotics. Clinical examination was unremarkable and the bladder was full. The cat was otherwise well.
i. What are your differential diagnoses?
   The only abnormality found on radiographic investigation is shown (4).
ii. What is your diagnosis and management advice for this case?

3 i. A soft tissue opacity is present in the caudodorsal thorax. Differential diagnoses include pleural or pulmonary disease, oesophageal disease or gastric herniation. After administration of liquid barium, the contrast material outlines rugal folds of the stomach within the thorax and a cranially displaced stomach in the abdomen consistent with a hiatal hernia.

ii. Hiatal hernias are usually congenital, but many dogs experience signs only intermittently due to the sliding nature of the stomach into the thorax from the abdomen. In dogs with minimal, only intermittent clinical signs, these may be best managed medically with H_2-blockers to control gastric acidity and reduce the common complication of oesophagitis. Prokinetic therapies and a low-fat diet may help to increase gastric motility and emptying. Surgical correction is required in animals with persistent signs of regurgitation and oesophageal disease.

4 i. Urinary tract infection; feline lower urinary tract disease (FLUTD)/feline urological syndrome (FUS); urinary tract calculi; urinary tract neoplasia; bleeding abnormalities; urinary tract trauma.

ii. The radiographic diagnosis is a single cystic calculus. The density of the stone suggests that the calculus is composed of struvite or oxalate. Provided other causes of haematuria have been excluded and any urinary tract infection identified, the treatment is surgical removal of the calculus via a cystotomy. The calculus should be analysed using a qualitative technique so that dietary changes or other relevant diagnostic tests can be performed to prevent recurrence. Urinalysis should be performed pre-operatively. In this case the calculus was composed of 100% calcium oxalate monohydrate. Advice was given to feed the cat a restricted protein, but not phosphate restricted, diet and monitor the urine, checking the pH and the presence of crystals. The possibility of an underlying hypercalcaemia was checked. The owners of this cat were warned that despite these measures recurrence could occur.

5 A ten-year-old, neutered male cat with diabetes mellitus was presented because of insulin resistance and bilaterally symmetric alopecia (5).
i. What are the possible causes of insulin resistance?
ii. What is the most likely diagnosis, and why?

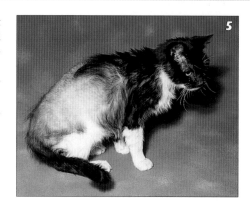

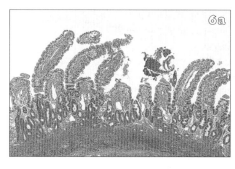

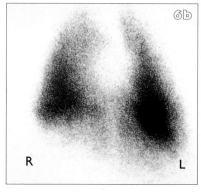

6 A six-year-old, neutered female Springer Spaniel suffering from chronic diarrhoea and weight loss suddenly develops ascites and dyspnoea. The dog has panhypoproteinaemia (albumin 13 g/l, globulin 12 g/l) and the ascitic fluid is a transudate. A protein-losing enteropathy is suspected and endoscopic biopsy ultimately confirms severe lymphocytic-plasmacytic enteritis (LPE) (6a). Chest radiographs reveal minimal pleural effusion, insufficient to explain the degree of dyspnoea exhibited by the patient. Although the lung parenchyma appears normal radiographically, a scintigraphic perfusion study is abnormal (6b); this indicates impaired pulmonary perfusion, especially of the caudal tip of the right caudal lung lobe.
i. What is the cause of the dyspnoea?
ii. How is it related to the enteropathy?

7 A seven-year-old, neutered female Springer Spaniel is diagnosed as having renal glomerulonephritis on a renal biopsy.
i. What are your treatment plans?
ii. What is the prognosis for dogs with glomerulonephritis?

5 i. Causes of apparent insulin resistance include infections, acromegaly, hyperthyroidism, exogenous glucocorticoid/progestogen administration, poor subcutaneous absorption of long-acting insulin preparations, and hyperadrenocorticism.

ii. Hyperadrenocorticism. Naturally occurring hyperadrenocorticism is a disease of middle-aged to old cats. Pituitary dependent hyperadrenocorticism and functional adrenal tumours have been described, although as in dogs the latter is less common. Cats appear to be peculiarly susceptible to the diabetogenic effects of chronic endogenous glucocorticoid excess and over 90% of cases present with concurrent diabetes mellitus. Hyperadrenocorticism should be suspected if other appropriate clinical signs are present. These include a pot-bellied appearance, alopecia of the trunk or ventral abdomen and, particularly in this species, thin atrophic skin which is fragile and easily torn with routine handling and grooming. Other clinical signs, e.g. polyuria/polydipsia and polyphagia, are attributable to the diabetic state. Almost all affected diabetic cats are poorly regulated with evidence of mild to severe insulin resistance.

6 i. Pulmonary thromboembolism. A scintigraphic perfusion study is performed by injecting ^{99m}technetium-labelled albumin microaggregates into the cephalic vein. The aggregates lodge in the first capillary bed they pass through (i.e. the pulmonary vasculature) and are detected by a gamma camera. All normally perfused lung will be visible scintigraphically but lack of perfusion will be indicated by a lack of scintillation. The lack of activity in the caudal tip of the left diaphragmatic is typical of a pulmonary thromboembolism. The absence of radiographic changes is expected and is the reason such a diagnosis is difficult to make routinely.

ii. Thromboembolism is a well recognized feature of the nephrotic syndrome, and is believed to be associated with the urinary loss of small anticoagulant factors, especially antithrombin III. Both pulmonary and renal thromboembolism are not infrequently reported at postmortem examination of dogs with protein-losing enteropathies, but are rarely diagnosed antemortem. The mechanism of thrombosis is presumably the same as for protein-losing nephropathies, and massive thrombosis may be an unexpected cause of death in these patients. As well as prednisolone and azathioprine treatment for the LPE, this dog was treated with heparin and low doses of aspirin, and it made a good recovery.

7 i. Remove, if possible, the inciting cause. Symptomatic and supportive therapy should be undertaken. Immunosuppressive drugs that may be tried include cyclophosphamide, azathioprine, corticosteroids and cyclosporin. Corticosteroids often result in worsening of the proteinuria and cyclosporin was not effective in one study; use of these drugs is less desirable. Drugs that decrease platelet aggregation, such as aspirin or dipyridamole, may be of benefit. Thromboxane synthetase inhibitors may help. Angiotensin converting enzyme (ACE) inhibitors may decrease the degree of proteinuria and reduce hypertension present in many cases. Monitor blood pressure as profound hypotension may develop where ACE inhibitors are used. Other supportive measures include feeding a low-sodium, low-protein diet. Beware of feeding a diet too low in protein as protein malnutrition may result due to excessive protein loss; serum albumin concentration should be monitored.

ii. As a general rule the prognosis is guarded at best.

8 An aged cat presents with an unkempt appearance, weight loss and polydipsia. Serum globulin concentration is 81 g/l; there are no other significant findings. Total thyroxine concentration is within the reference range and the feline coronavirus titre is negative. The haematological profile and a photomicrograph of the blood film (8) are shown.

i. What do you observe in the photomicrograph?
ii. Can you explain the findings?
iii. How do you interpret this haematological profile?
iv. What would be your next step towards a diagnosis?

RBCs ($\times 10^{12}$/l)	4.7
Hb (g/l)	70
PCV (l/l)	0.33
MCV (fl)	70
MCHC (g/l)	220
nRBCs	0%
WBCs ($\times 10^9$/l)	3.6
Neutrophils (seg) ($\times 10^9$/l)	3.28
Neutrophils (bands) ($\times 10^9$/l)	0
Lymphocytes ($\times 10^9$/l)	0.11
Monocytes ($\times 10^9$/l)	0.14
Eosinophils ($\times 10^9$/l)	0.07

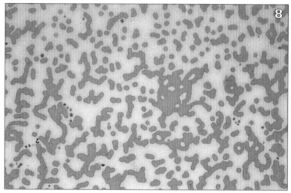

9 Your client has four cats ranging from one to four years of age and you have tested them for FeLV using an ELISA assay for FeLV antigen. Two cats are FeLV positive.
What advice would you give to your client?

8 i. The RBCs are agglutinated, there is no evidence of polychromasia or anisocytosis, and the platelet count appears adequate.

ii. This is a non-regenerative anaemia with autoagglutination. The agglutination is probably secondary to the elevated globulin concentration. Presumably there are antibodies present with RBC specificity/cross-reactivity.

iii. This is a mild non-regenerative anaemia. The sample was sent to a laboratory and the elevated MCV is either due to RBC swelling or use of an automatic analyser calibrated for human RBCs rather than feline RBCs. The artefactually elevated MCV has also erroneously elevated the PCV. There is a lymphopenia with a low-normal neutrophil count. The overall findings are suspicious of bone marrow suppression/disease.

iv. The findings to date are suspicious for multiple myeloma, lymphoma/leukaemia or possibly another neoplasm. Protein electrophoresis followed by bone marrow biopsy would be indicated. This case showed a monoclonal gamma globulin spike and had increased plasma cells on aspiration of the bone marrow, confirming the diagnosis of myeloma.

9 The positive cats may fit into any of the following scenarios (in descending order of likelihood):

- They may be truly FeLV positive, 85% of whom will be dead within 3.5 years.
- The result may be a false positive. FeLV positive results derived from ELISA or rapid immunomigration (RIM) tests should be confirmed by virus isolation (VI) or immunofluorescent assay (IFA), especially in healthy cats.
- The cat may be in the very short period between infection and development of immunity. In this case, retest after 12 weeks. If the cat is still FeLV positive, then it will remain positive.
- They may be positive by ELISA or RIM and negative by VI or IFA. Discordant cats are difficult to manage; the best one can do is to keep retesting them every 1–3 months. Around half of discordant cats eventually become negative by both tests, some become positive on both tests and others remain discordant almost indefinitely. Discordant cats may be latently infected and do not appear to be infectious to other cats unless they become positive by VI, at which time they are then infectious.

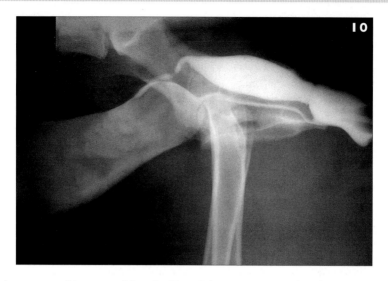

10 A two-year-old, neutered female Giant Schnauzer presented with urinary incontinence of several months' duration. The dog leaked when recumbent and the severity of the incontinence varied. The dog was otherwise normal. She was spayed at 11 months old after her first season and was not incontinent as a puppy.

i. How would you investigate this dog?

This radiograph was obtained (10).

ii. What is your main differential diagnosis?

11 A six-year-old Labrador stud dog unsuccessfully mated three bitches over the last six months. He has previously been fertile. He has normal libido and is not ill. His total spermatozoal output is normal but spermatozoal motility is reduced. A smear of the semen has been stained with nigrosin and eosin (11).

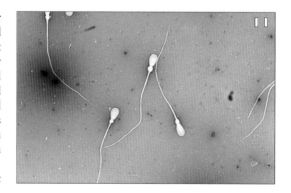

i. What is the predominant spermatozoal abnormality?

ii. What is the significance of these changes?

iii. What is the likely aetiology of this condition?

iv. What is the prognosis for a return to fertility?

10 i. • Full clinical examination with specific reference to the urinary and nervous system.
• Urine collected by cystocentesis or catheterization for bacteriology and urinalysis.
• Blood for routine haematology and biochemistry.
• Plain radiographic (lateral and ventrodorsal) examination of the abdomen after suitable preparation (enemas should be given to remove faeces from the rectum).
• Intravenous urogram. Give 700 mg/kg iodine via the cephalic vein with ventrodorsal views taken at 0 and 5 minutes and lateral views of the abdomen and caudal abdomen taken at 10 and 15 minutes respectively. A small amount of air introduced into the bladder prior to injection of contrast improves visualization of the ureterovesical terminations.
• Retrograde vagino-urethrogram. Allows accurate determination of the position of the bladder neck and may confirm the presence and morphology of an ectopic ureter.
• Ultrasound examination of the bladder after residual air and contrast has been removed and the bladder moderately filled with sterile saline. This allows identification of ureterovesical junctions and visualization of ureteral jets from ureters entering the trigone normally. Alternatively, direct visualization of ureteral emptying with fluoroscopy.
• Urodynamic investigation. Stressed urethral pressure profilometry is a better predictor of continence than plain urethral pressure profilometry. Both techniques require expensive equipment and are dependent upon the technique used. Urethral pressure profilometry can provide additional useful information.
ii. In this case the history, lack of specific findings on clinical and radiographic examinations, and presence of an intrapelvic bladder neck on the radiograph were highly suggestive of urethral sphincter mechanism incompetence. The dog responded well to treatment with phenylpropanolamine and subsequent colposuspension. Other common causes of urinary incontinence were ruled out by the above investigation.

11 i. Nigrosin–eosin staining of semen is useful since it allows the differentiation of live (white) from dead (pink) spermatozoa. In this slide all the spermatozoa are live and each demonstrates a similar morphological abnormality located on the mid-piece region. There is swelling of the proximal mid-piece. These defects may be described as proximal cytoplasmic droplets; in this case the lesions are not completely regular in shape or size and are more accurately termed proximal mid-piece swellings.
ii. Spermatozoa with proximal mid-piece swellings frequently have poor motility, since this region is packed with mitochondria and provides propulsive force to the tail. Electron microscopic studies of these spermatozoa usually show axonemal and mitochondrial defects accounting for the poor motility, as well as other membrane defects. The latter are presumably the reason why these spermatozoa are infertile.
iii. The aetiology of these defects is uncertain; however, it is clear that they are primary spermatozoa abnormalities, i.e. they occur during spermatogenesis. Proximal mid-piece swellings are commonly found in aged infertile dogs and there is some evidence of the condition being found with a high frequency in certain breeds.
iv. In most cases the prognosis for fertility is hopeless and hormonal therapies are unrewarding.

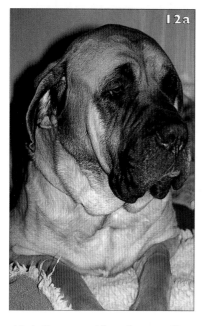

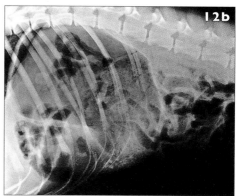

12 A five-year-old, male Mastiff (**12a**) presents to your emergency service retching and collapsed, with a large tympanic abdomen, one hour after his morning meal. A lateral abdominal radiograph is obtained (**12b**).
i. What is your radiographic diagnosis?
ii. What medical therapy will you recommend?
iii. Is surgery indicated? If so, what preventive measures might you perform to avoid a recurrence?

13 A six-year-old Yorkshire Terrier with profuse chronic diarrhoea is diagnosed on intestinal biopsy as having lymphangiectasia (**13**).
i. What is intestinal lymphangiectasia, and what is its cause(s)?
ii. What changes might be found on haematological and serum biochemical evaluation?
iii. How is intestinal lymphangiectasia treated?

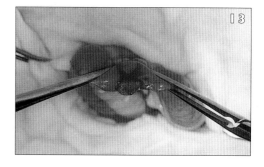

12 i. The stomach is severely distended with gas, there is compartmentalization of the gas ('double bubble') and the duodenum is dislocated cranially indicating the presence of a gastric torsion.

ii. Gastric torsions are true medical emergencies and require aggressive intervention with gastric decompression, treatment of shock with fluids, and correction of acid-base status and cardiac dysrhythmias. An attempt should be made to pass a tube into the stomach and, if this is unsuccessful, a trocar may be necessary to relieve acute gaseous distension. A large-bore intravenous catheter should be placed to allow for rapid fluid administration and correction of blood gas and electrolyte derangements which occur secondary to the sequestration of acids in the stomach and increased intra-abdominal pressures. A continuous ECG is useful to assess for the presence of and/or response to therapy for cardiac dysrhythmias.

iii. Surgery is indicated as soon as the animal is sufficiently stabilized to undergo anaesthesia. Surgical intervention has three goals; to reposition the stomach and spleen, assess organ viability, and perform a gastropexy to discourage recurrences.

13 i. Dilation of the lacteals of the villi and submucosal lymphatics. Lymphatic dilatation may be secondary to a proximal obstruction, but is more commonly idiopathic. It can be associated with lipogranuloma formation in the mesentery; this is thought to be a response to leakage of chyle into the tissue.

ii. Lymphangiectasia is one cause of a protein-losing enteropathy with hypoalbuminaemia and hypoglobulinaemia occurring. Leakage of lymph into the gut lumen results in loss of cholesterol and lymphocytes, with consequent hypocholesterolaemia and lymphopenia.

iii. Feed a severely fat-restricted diet. Medium chain triglycerides can be given as a fat source as they are absorbed directly into the portal blood and not via the lymphatics. Steroid administration is beneficial in some cases, either because of associated lymphangitis/lipogranulomas or because of an incorrect diagnosis. Lymphocytic-plasmacytic enteritis is occasionally misdiagnosed as lymphangiectasia because of lacteal dilatation associated with lamina propria infiltration.

14 A five-year-old, neutered female cat presented with clinical signs of diabetes mellitus despite administration of 15 iu of a purified beef lente insulin once daily over the previous ten months. Following the owner's regimen of insulin injection and *ad lib* feeding, two-hourly blood glucose concentrations were measured over a 24 hour period (**14**).

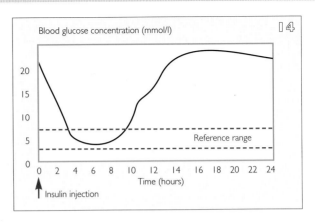

i. What is your diagnosis?
ii. How should the treatment be altered?
iii. What other diagnostic test is useful in monitoring long-term glycaemic control?

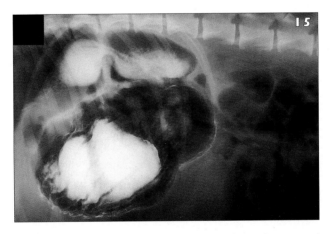

15 This radiograph (**15**) was taken of an Irish Wolfhound presented with acute vomiting and collapse of a few hours' duration. The dog's mucous membranes were dark, a tachycardia was present and the abdomen was enlarged and tense. Percussion of the cranial abdomen resulted in tympany. An ECG showed a ventricular tachyarrhythmia with numerous ventricular ectopics.
i. What is your diagnosis?
ii. How would you consider feeding this dog postoperatively?

14 i. There is a short duration of insulin effect. Based on the glucose concentrations, the insulin appears to have a duration of effect of approximately ten hours. The concentrations do not fall below the reference range at any time thus precluding a diagnosis of Somogyi overswing (posthypoglycaemia rebound hyperglycaemia). Insulins are categorized as short-acting (regular/semi-lente), intermediate-acting (isophane (NPH)/lente) or long-acting (protamine zinc (PZI) ultralente). Blood glucose concentrations in diabetic cats are rarely controlled for longer than 12 hours after injection of NPH or lente insulins because of rapid metabolism of the insulin. NPH and lente insulin have an onset of activity of approximately 30 minutes; insulin concentrations peak at approximately 90 minutes and subsequently fall to basal values at approximately eight hours. PZI and ultralente insulin preparations have a longer duration of effect but are less potent.

ii. Changing the frequency of injection, or type or dose of insulin. The animal should be re-stabilized using either the lente insulin twice daily or substitution with a long-acting preparation; once daily injections of a long-acting preparation may require higher doses. Further adjustments in dose or frequency of administration should be made based on the clinical response to therapy and serial blood glucose curves.

iii. Measurement of serum fructosamine concentrations. Fructosamine is a glycated protein whose concentration is largely dependent on the mean glucose concentration over the preceding 1–3 weeks. Serum fructosamine concentrations are easily measured using an automated colorimetric assay available in most commercial laboratories. In this case, measurement of a single blood glucose concentration between two and eight hours after insulin injection would provide a false impression of adequate glycaemic control. Concurrent measurement of a serum fructosamine concentration would have confirmed the clinical suspicions of a poorly regulated diabetic state.

15 i. The radiograph shows a dilated torsed stomach. There is compartmentalization of the gas and the soft tissue 'cross' seen within the gastric silhouette is characteristic of gastric torsion. The duodenum is displaced dorsally.

ii. If the stomach wall is relatively healthy, feeding through a gastrostomy tube, nasal feeding tube or by mouth would suffice. The benefit of feeding through a gastrostomy tube or oesophageal tube is that the risk of redilation immediately postoperatively is removed. If there is extensive necrosis of the stomach wall, nil by mouth is indicated and feeding using total parenteral nutrition (TPN) or partial parenteral nutrition (PPN) should be instituted. PPN has the advantage that it is cheaper and can be provided through a peripheral catheter, in contrast to TPN which must be administered into the cranial vena cava. The disadvantage with PPN is that only some of the dog's nutritional needs can be met and thus it is only suitable for short-term use.

		Antibody titre a	Antibody titre b
CCV	Pup 1	1:2	1:128
	Pup 2	1:4	1:256
	Pup 3	1:2	1:64
CPV	Pup 1	1:320	1:160
	Pup 2	1:160	1:320
	Pup 3	1:160	1:80
CDV	Pup 1	1:400	1:200
	Pup 2	1:200	1:200
	Pup 3	1:200	1:100
(Titre a at presentation, titre b two weeks after presentation)			

16 A ten-week-old litter of pups is presented with acute diarrhoea and inappetence. The pups are bright and vomiting is not a feature. No blood or mucus is present in the faeces. The bitch had been vaccinated against canine parvovirus (CPV) and canine distemper virus (CDV) eight months previously. Faecal analysis for protozoae, worm eggs and coccidia was negative. Faecal streptococci and non-haemolytic *E. coli* were isolated from the faeces. The results of CDV, CPV and canine coronavirus (CCV) serology in three of the affected pups at the time of presentation (a) and two weeks later (b) are shown.

i. How would you interpret these results?
ii. Could you confirm your diagnosis?

17 You are presented with a three-year-old maiden Labrador bitch that has had a serosanguinous vulval discharge for 12 days. The owners wish to breed from her but she has refused to stand for the male on the past two days. A vaginal smear has been obtained and stained with a modified Wright-Giemsa stain (**17**).

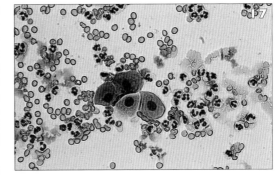

i. What cell types are present in this vaginal smear?
ii. What is the stage of the oestrous cycle?
iii. Why has mating been refused?
iv. How can this problem be overcome?

16 i. The rise in antibody titres to CCV is consistent with the presence of an active infection, whereas the antibody titres to CPV and CDV show no significant change. The other results provide no evidence for any other infectious agent.

ii. Confirmation of CCV infection is difficult. Virus isolation may be attempted on fresh samples. However, the virus is labile in the environment and some strains do not adapt well to cell culture systems. Electron microscopy is useful in that live CCV does not need to be present. However, with storage the characteristic club-like projections associated with CCV are lost, making recognition of the virus difficult. Histopathological examination of the small intestine is not helpful as there are no characteristic changes recognized. Immunohistochemical staining for CCV antigen would be helpful.

17 i. Small intermediate epithelial cells (clustered in the centre of the field of view), red blood cells and numerous neutrophils. Amorphous cellular debris is also abundant.

ii. In view of the large number of neutrophils it is likely that the bitch has entered metoestrus (dioestrus). This stage of the oestrous cycle is characterized by a decrease in the percentage of anuclear and large intermediate epithelial cells in the vaginal smear, and an increase in cellular debris associated with sloughing of the vaginal mucosa. Metoestrus is also associated with an influx of neutrophils in large numbers. These cells have been excluded from the vaginal lumen during oestrus due to proliferation of the vaginal mucosa.

iii. The onset of metoestrus is associated with a rise in plasma progesterone concentrations which causes the termination of oestrus; behavioural signs of oestrus are therefore absent. Most owners consider that the optimum mating time is between ten and 14 days from the onset of proestrus. However, this is not always the case and many bitches ovulate soon after the onset of proestrus (as early as day 5 – as in the present case), while others may not ovulate until much later (sometimes as late as day 30).

iv. This bitch has a relatively short proestrus but is normal. The problem is the result of a misunderstanding of normal reproductive physiology. The optimum time of mating cannot be calculated simply by counting the number of days from the onset of proestrus. More accurate assessments of the optimal mating time include the evaluation of vaginal exfoliative cytology, vaginal endoscopy and the measurement of plasma progesterone concentrations using an ELISA test kit. **NB:** Evaluate each oestrous period independently.

18 An 18-month-old domestic shorthair cat is presented with dyspnoea and inappetence. There is no history of polydipsia/polyuria or of CNS signs. On thoracic auscultation lung and heart sounds are muffled; no murmur is audible. Respiratory rate is 40 breaths/minute and the pulse rate 160 bpm. Mucous membranes are unremarkable and capillary refill time normal. Abdominal palpation shows no abnormality. No lymphadenopathy is present and examination of the eye is unremarkable. A dorsoventral radiograph of the chest shows the heart shadow to be obscured by a thoracic effusion.

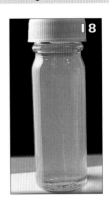

i. List the possible causes of thoracic effusion in the cat, and describe the fluid that you may obtain on thoracocentesis in each of the examples you have listed.

Thoracocentesis produces this fluid (**18**).

ii. What tests will you perform on the fluid, and what are you looking for?

iii. What virological tests will you do on the blood/effusion?

iv. Suppose the blood tests you did were negative; is your diagnosis necessarily wrong?

v. What else can you do to confirm your diagnosis?

19 Two photomicrographs of centrifuged sediments from abdominal effusions in middle-aged cats are shown (**19a, 19b**). They are stained with Wright's stain. One is from a chyloabdomen and the other from a case of FIP.

i. Which is which, and why?

ii. How would you describe the appearance of the macrophages in both photomicrographs?

iii. How do you confirm that a fluid is chylous?

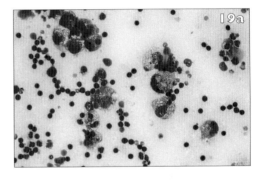

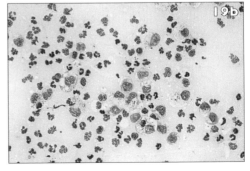

18 i. • Thymic lymphoma: serous transudate (clear, watery), serosanguinous exudate (blood tinged) or a chylous effusion (milky).
• FIP: exudate – (clear, yellowish), froths on shaking; may clot.
• Cardiomyopathy: transudate (clear, thin, watery).
• Pyothorax: pus, exudate (thick, yellow) foul smelling.
• Ruptured thoracic duct: chyle (milky or pink), high in triglycerides.
• *Aelurostrongylus abstrusus* infection: serous transudate (clear, watery).
• Diaphragmatic hernia: serous transudate (clear, watery).
ii. Cytology:
• Thymic lymphoma: tumour cells (lymphocytes) are often present.
• FIP: non-degenerate neutrophils and macrophages with a cell count of <5,000 cells/ml.
• Ruptured diaphragm, cardiomyopathy: low cellularity, few non-degenerate neutrophils and macrophages.
• *Aelurostrongylus abstrusus*: larvae in a tracheal wash which have a characteristic S-shaped kink in the tail.
Biochemistry:
• Total protein: exudates >35 g/l; transudates <35 g/l. In FIP the total protein is likely to be >35 g/l.
• Albumin:globulin ratio: if <0.45, FIP is very likely; if >0.8, FIP is very unlikely; if between 0.4 and 0.8, FIP is possible.
iii. FeLV antigen: 90+% of thymic lymphomas are FeLV-related; FIP antibody titre.
iv. No. FeLV negativity does not rule out a diagnosis of thymic lymphoma. Occasionally, cats with effusive FIP are seronegative on standard antibody tests because there is so much virus that it combines with all the antibody, leaving none available for the test.
v. Needle biopsy of the tumour will confirm the diagnosis of thymic lymphoma. In the case of antibody test negative FIP, detection of feline coronavirus in the effusion is required.

19 i. 19a is the chyloabdomen. The presence of small lymphocytes and foamy (fat-filled/active) macrophages is suggestive of fatty lymph/chyle. **19b** is FIP. Note the blue background staining of the high-protein effusion, foamy (protein-filled/active) macrophages and neutrophils. Small lymphocytes are quite uncommon in effusions associated with FIP.
ii. These are active foamy macrophages.
iii. Biochemical analysis showing a greater triglyceride concentration in the fluid than in serum confirms that a fluid is chylous.

20 This abdominal radiograph (**20**) was obtained in a two-year-old, female black Standard Poodle with gradual abdominal enlargement, depression and anorexia. On physical examination the dog was thin and jaundiced, and had ascites. Rectal examination revealed melena. Clinical pathology show-ed a mildly regenerative

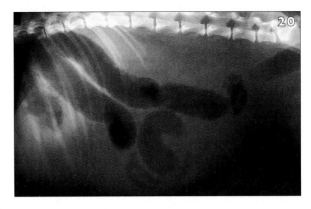

anaemia (PCV 0.25 l/l), hypoproteinaemia (albumin 16 g/l, globulin 22 g/l), elevated liver enzymes (ALP 526 u/l, ALT 456 u/l) and high bilirubin concentration (102 µmol/l).

i. What comments can you make on the radiograph?
ii. How can you explain the melena, and how should you treat it?
iii. Should you biopsy the liver in this dog?

21 An Irish Setter is presented with a peripheral lymphadenopathy involving the submandibular (**21**), prescapular, inguinal, axillary and popliteal lymph nodes. As far as the owner is concerned the dog is otherwise unremarkable, bright, eating and drinking normally. On physical examination no abnormalities other than the lymphadenopathy are recognized.

i. What are the main differential diagnoses to consider?
ii. How might you confirm the diagnosis?
iii. What serum biochemical tests might you be interested in performing?

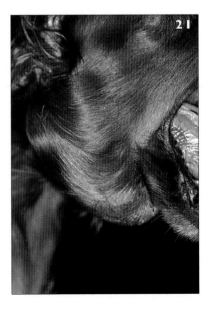

20 i. The radiograph shows reduced detail compatible with ascites. The liver is small, which suggests chronic liver disease.

ii. Liver disease and portal hypertension often cause GI ulceration due to gastric acid hypersecretion, impaired gastric mucosal blood flow and/or reduced epithelial cell turnover. GI blood loss may explain the anaemia and hypoproteinaemia; the latter may also be due to portal hypertension causing renal water retention and haemodilution. Since GI bleeding may precipitate hepatic encephalopathy, treatment with H_2 blockers (e.g. famotidine 0.5 mg/kg q24h) and/or sucralfate (0.5–1.0 gm q8h) is advocated. Cimetidine is not recommended.

Dogs with severe liver disease may have coagulopathies due to decreased production of clotting factors and/or disseminated intravascular coagulation (DIC). Reduced production of clotting factors usually produces a subclinical coagulopathy, which may result in bleeding after invasive medical procedures. A coagulation screen may show abnormalities suggestive of DIC such as thrombocytopenia, prolonged prothrombin/thromboplastin times and increased fibrin degradation products. Treatment with plasma and/or heparin may be given, but the prognosis is poor.

iii. Jaundice, ascites and small liver size suggest chronic liver disease. A liver biopsy should be taken for exact diagnosis and prognosis. It is important to distinguish between chronic hepatitis, which is medically manageable, and cirrhosis, which is end-stage liver disease and has a poor prognosis. Coagulation should be assessed prior to biopsy. Pretreatment with parenteral vitamin K1 (2 mg/kg q12h for 2 days) is recommended in case of a subclinical coagulopathy.

21 i. Lymph node enlargement may arise as a consequence of proliferation of the normal cells (a reactive lymph node), infiltration with inflammatory cells (lymphadenitis) or infiltration with neoplastic cells. In this case a generalized bacterial lymphadenitis would be unlikely given the lack of signs of ill health. Reactive lymph nodes may arise as a result of antigenic stimulation following an infectious or inflammatory disorder and cannot be ruled out in this case. However, the commonest cause of a generalized lymphadenopathy is lymphoma, which comprise 80% or more of cases.

ii. The diagnosis may be confirmed with a fine-needle aspirate or lymph node biopsy. Avoid the submandibular lymph node if possible, as this node often has a reactive appearance because it drains the oral cavity, and misdiagnosis is therefore possible.

iii. Lymphoma may involve any organ system. Thus, assessment of liver enzymes and liver function (e.g. bile acids) and renal parameters (urea and creatinine) are indicated. In addition, assessment of calcium, phosphate, albumin and globulin are indicated as hypercalcaemia and hyperglobulinaemia may develop as paraneoplastic processes.

22 This five-month-old domestic shorthair cat has a history of reduced appetite and poor growth since it was obtained by the owners as a kitten. More recently the cat had intermittent episodes of hyperactive behaviour alternating with lethargy. The owners further report that the cat often salivates excessively. On physical examination the cat is found to be in poor body condition and the kidneys feel prominent on abdominal palpation.

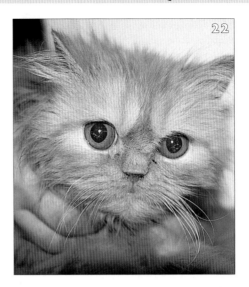

i. What do you observe in the illustration (22)?
ii. What is the differential diagnosis?
iii. How would you establish the diagnosis?

23 A ten-year-old, neutered male cat with diabetes mellitus presented because of insulin resistance, a pot-bellied appearance and bilaterally symmetric alopecia. Haematology was unremarkable. Serum biochemistry showed a mild increase in cholesterol, ALT and ALP. Urinalysis showed SG of 1.040 and +++ glucose on a dipstick.
i. What condition do you suspect?
ii. What laboratory tests are most useful in confirming a diagnosis?
iii. What treatment options exist?

24 A free-ranging cat is presented in the autumn with scabs around the face and right forepaw.
i. You suspect cat pox infection. How will you confirm your diagnosis?
ii. You consider treating the cat symptomatically while awaiting the laboratory results. Will you use corticosteroids?
iii. What advice will you give to the owner about handling the cat?

22 i. Copper-coloured irises, a common but unexplained finding in cats with congenital portosystemic shunts.

ii. Behavioural changes may result from metabolic or CNS diseases. The intermittency of the signs is most compatible with metabolic disease, such as hepatic or uraemic encephalopathy, hypoglycaemia, hypocalcaemia and lead intoxication. Hepatic encephalopathy due to a congenital portosystemic shunt is the commonest cause of intermittent neurobehavioural signs in young cats. Signs include hypersalivation, depression, behaviour changes, head pressing, apparent blindness and seizures. Renal enlargement may occur, probably attributable to compensatory hypertrophy.

iii. Laboratory tests can rule out metabolic encephalopathies. In cats with congenital portosystemic shunts, liver enzymes can be moderately increased and RBC microcytosis may be present. Fasting serum bile acids are usually high but are occasionally normal. Postprandial bile acids (obtained two hours after feeding) are always increased. Elevated blood ammonia signifies hepatic encephalopathy; normal levels do not rule it out. Radiography usually shows a small liver and occasionally large kidneys. Ultrasonography may identify the shunting vessel. Rectal portal scintigraphy is a non-invasive technique for detection of shunts, but since it requires radioactivity its use is limited to referral centres. Definitive diagnosis is often based on mesenteric portography.

23 i. Hyperadrenocorticism (HAC).

ii. Leucocytosis, eosinopenia, lymphopenia and monocytosis are inconsistent findings with HAC. Biochemical abnormalities, including hypercholesterolaemia, high ALT and, less commonly, ALP activities, relate in part to the diabetic state. Cats do not have a specific steroid-induced ALP isoenzyme. Isosthenuric urine is rarely documented.

Adrenal function tests are indicated as basal serum cortisol concentrations are of little diagnostic value. A combination of an exaggerated cortisol response to exogenous ACTH administration and a lack of suppression after high-dose dexamethasone administration appear to be the most useful methods of distinguishing cases of HAC from healthy animals or those with non-adrenal illness. False positive and false negative results occur; they should be interpreted in the light of the clinical findings.

iii. Surgical adrenalectomy is the treatment of choice for functional adrenal tumours and is also recommended for pituitary dependent HAC. Medical management with op'-DDD (mitotane) or ketoconazole is unrewarding. Management with metyrapone has shown promise in some cats but is not readily available. Cobalt-60 irradiation for visible pituitary tumours has been used with partial success in a few cats but is of limited availability and is a major expense. Insulin requirements can drop precipitously if the hyperadrenocorticism is successfully treated.

24 i. By sending a scab in a sterile container to a laboratory for virus isolation.

ii. Corticosteroids are absolutely contraindicated in cat pox infection; they can cause the virus to become systemic, with lethal effects.

iii. Cat pox is potentially a zoonotic infection, so the owners should be advised to take extra careful hygienic precautions when handling the cat.

25 This eight-year-old, entire male Jack Russell Terrier presented with a two-month history of progressive vomiting and abnormal posturing. The owner reported that when the dog first became ill he would eat normally and vomit perhaps once or twice a week. However, in recent weeks he has been vomiting more frequently, up to three times daily. He is now inappetent and is often seen in the stance shown (25a), with his forelimbs and sternum touching the floor and his back end elevated. Routine haematology reveals a mild non-regenerative anaemia (PCV 0.32 l/l). No abnormalities are apparent on a biochemical profile or abdominal radiograph.

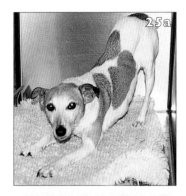

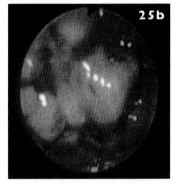

i. What clinical conditions are associated with this particular body posture?
ii. What diagnostic tests may help you reach a definitive diagnosis?
iii. Describe what you see in the endoscopic view of the fundus of the stomach in this dog (25b). List your differential diagnoses.

26 A ten-year-old, female Cairn Terrier presents with polydipsia, polyuria, weight gain and exercise intolerance of four weeks' duration. The caudal edge of the liver is palpable beyond the costochondral junction. Pertinent biochemical abnormalities include increased serum liver enzyme activities

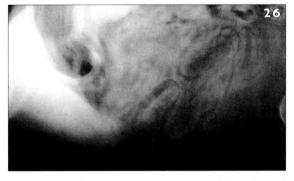

(ALT 234 u/l, ALP 2,398 u/l) and a hypercholesterolaemia (13.8 mmol/l). A lateral abdominal radiograph is taken (26).
i. Describe the radiographic abnormalities.
ii. Discuss a list of differential diagnoses.
iii. What further diagnostic tests might be indicated?

25 i. This body posture is referred to as the 'praying mantis position' or the 'position of relief'. Dogs suffering from cranial abdominal pain will assume this position which is thought to relieve pressure in the abdomen. Causes of cranial abdominal pain include pancreatitis, gastric inflammation, distension, ulcers, foreign bodies, neoplasia, peritonitis, or, less frequently, other infectious or inflammatory diseases involving the liver, kidney or GI tract.

ii. Since pancreatitis is a common cause of abdominal pain, further laboratory investigations such as serum amylase, lipase and trypsin-like immunoreactivity (TLI) assays may prove helpful. Imaging studies such as abdominal ultrasound may allow direct visualization of pancreatic inflammation, masses, intestinal wall thickenings or peritoneal effusions. This is not always sensitive when evaluating gastric disease. Contrast radiographic studies such as feeding barium meals may outline masses, foreign material, wall thickenings or ulcers within the stomach and small intestine. Endoscopy of the upper GI tract is highly sensitive in evaluating for gastric and small intestinal mucosal disease.

iii. There is a large, lobulated mass in the fundus of the stomach, covered superficially by normal appearing gastric mucosa. There is no ulceration evident; however, other areas revealed ulcerated mucosa and the dark material on the surface of this mass suggests the presence of digested blood. Chronic blood loss and subsequent iron deficiency may account for the low-grade, non-regenerative anaemia. The mass obliterated the body of the fundus, obstructing the pyloric outflow tract and making resection difficult and unlikely to be successful. Gastric neoplasias are infrequent in the dog. They may be benign (e.g. polyps or leiomyomas), malignant (e.g. lymphosarcoma, adenocarcinoma, leiomyosarcoma or fibrosarcoma) or, rarely, metastatic in origin. This mass was an adenocarcinoma.

26 i. The liver is seen to extend caudally well beyond the costochondral junction, with a rounded caudal edge.

ii. The hepatomegaly as seen radiographically appears to be diffuse as evidenced by the caudal displacement of abdominal contents and rounded liver margins. Hepatomegaly may be a result of congestion, as in congestive heart failure, or infiltration with inflammatory cells (hepatitis), neoplastic cells (lymphoma) or cellular accumulation of lipid (diabetes mellitus), glycogen (hyperadrenocorticism) or excess metabolites (congenital storage diseases). The history and biochemical findings in this dog are suggestive of hyperadrenocorticism.

iii. An ultrasound examination of the liver and adrenals helps to further define the extent and nature of the disease. With a high suspicion of hyperadrenocorticism, testing of adrenal function is an appropriate next step. A fine-needle aspirate or biopsy of the liver may aid in characterizing any suspected infiltrative diseases. In this dog a diffuse hyperechogenic liver and the appearance of vacuolated hepatocytes on cytology is consistent with a steroid hepatopathy and supportive of the diagnosis of hyperadrenocorticism.

27 A seven-year-old, neutered female Springer Spaniel presented for evaluation of polyuria and polydipsia. Physical examination was unremarkable. Laboratory evaluation is shown. Heartworm antigen test was negative. Serum antibody titres for borreliosis, Rocky Mountain spotted fever, ehrlichiosis and leptospirosis were negative. ANA titre 1:128. Rare LE cells were present. Urine cytology revealed struvite crystals only. Antithrombin III was found to be 51% of normal.
i. What is your interpretation of these data?
ii. Would you perform a renal biopsy?
iii. Describe techniques for performing renal biopsy.

Albumin (g/l)	21
ALP (u/l)	36
Total protein (g/l)	43
Urea (mmol/l)	6.8
Creatinine (μmol/l)	80
Glucose (mmol/l)	5.9
Sodium (mmol/l)	148
Potassium (mmol/l)	4.6
Chloride (mmol/l)	117
Calcium (mmol/l)	2.1
Phosphorus (mmol/l)	1.4
PCV (l/l)	0.49
WBCs ($\times$ 10^9/l)	8.2
Platelet ($\times$ 10^9/l)	313

White cell differential unremarkable.
Urinalysis:

Colour/turbidity	Yellow/cloudy
SG	1.014
Glucose, ketones, bilirubin, occult blood	Negative
Protein (mg/dl)	1,604
Creatinine (mg/dl)	234

28 A four-year-old, female German Shepherd Dog is presented with a large swelling protruding from the vulval lips (**28**). The bitch commenced proestrus ten days previously and presently has a serosanginous discharge and is attractive to male dogs.
i. What are the differential diagnoses?
ii. What is the aetiology of this condition?
iii. What will happen if this condition is untreated?
iv. What treatment options are available?

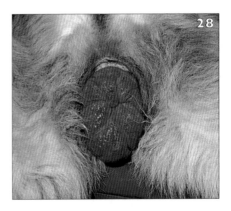

27 i. The urine SG is consistent with a polyuric state. However, it may also represent recent ingestion of water. More significant is the 4+ proteinuria with a SG of 1.014. This is probably a real finding because the serum albumin concentration is also low. As there is no indication of haematuria, pyuria or bacteriuria on examination of urine sediment, the proteinuria is probably significant and should be evaluated further. In order to determine if the proteinuria is significant the urine protein:creatinine ratio (UP:C) should be calculated. This is technically easier to perform than quantification of 24 hour urine protein excretion. The UP:C ratio in this dog is 6.85:1 which is significantly elevated.

Significant proteinuria not associated with haematuria, pyuria or bacteriuria is usually glomerular in origin. Causes of glomerular proteinuria may be investigated through testing the immune system, evaluating for infectious diseases and renal biopsy. The moderately high ANA titre is consistent with an immunological cause, e.g. systemic lupus erythematosus. The low antithrombin III reflects loss of this compound through the leaky glomeruli.

ii. Yes. A renal biopsy is still indicated to distinguish between glomerulonephritis and amyloidosis.

iii. There are several techniques for renal biopsy:
• A surgical biopsy may be obtained via laparotomy.
• A biopsy may be obtained percutaneously using ultrasound guidance.
• A key hole technique may be employed to obtain a biopsy of the right kidney.

28 i. Vaginal hyperplasia protruding through the vulval lips. Other differential diagnoses include protrusion of a vaginal tumour or polyp and vaginal/uterine prolapse. The latter is very rare and usually only occurs post partum. Palpation of the protruding tissue demonstrates that it originates from the vaginal wall cranial to the external urethral orifice, involving the whole circumference of the vagina rather than the ventral vaginal floor. Vaginal hyperplasia occurs almost solely during proestrus and oestrus and often recurs cyclically.

ii. Hyperplasia of the vaginal mucosa occurs in response to elevation of plasma oestrogen concentration. The hyperplastic tissue develops from the vaginal floor cranial to the urethral orifice, but as the condition progresses (and often worsens) the tissue may involve the circumference of the vagina. The increase in size causes it to protrude through the vulval lips.

iii. In all cases the hyperplastic vaginal mucosa regresses at the onset of metoestrus when oestrogen concentrations decrease and progesterone concentrations increase. Provided that the tissue is not traumatized and does not desiccate, it will return to normal within a few weeks. Bitches that become pregnant do not have difficulty at parturition since the hyperplastic tissue is not present at this time.

iv. In the majority of cases only conservative treatment is warranted and the application of emollient creams and the prevention of self-trauma is sufficient. If the tissue is traumatized or the animal is required for breeding, a submucosal resection via an episiotomy may be necessary. Surgery can be avoided by the use of artificial insemination where allowed. Serious consideration should be given to not breeding from affected animals.

29 A six-year-old, female West Highland White Terrier is presented with a peracute history of depression and vomiting. The dog is hypothermic (37.3°C [99.2°F]) and haemorrhagic diarrhoea is found on the thermometer. The results of routine blood work are shown.

i. What is your presumptive diagnosis, and why?
ii. How would you treat this animal?
iii. What is the prognosis?

PCV (l/l)	0.79
Platelets (× 10⁹/l)	155
WBCs (× 10⁹/l)	12.1
Differential white cell count	Unremarkable
Total protein (g/l)	70
Albumin (g/l)	34
Globulin (g/l)	36
Sodium (mmol/l)	155
Potassium (mmol/l)	4.5
Urea (mmol/l)	8
Creatinine (µmol/l)	105
ALT (u/l)	105
ALP (u/l)	86

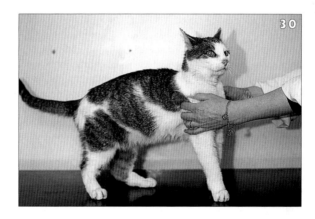

30 An eight-year-old, neutered female cat presented because of mild weight loss and intermittent diarrhoea over the preceding four weeks (30). The only abnormality noted was a small left cervical nodule.
i. What is the most likely diagnosis?
ii. What is the cause of this condition?
   Thyroid hormone analyses gave the following results: total thyroxine (T4) – 84.2 nmol/l; total triiodothyronine (T3) – 0.72 nmol/l.
iii. How would you interpret these results?
iv. What other clinical signs may be seen with this condition?

29 & 30: Answers

29 i. Haemorrhagic gastroenteritis (HGE). This condition typically affects small dogs (including Yorkshire, Maltese, Cairn and West Highland White Terriers, and Miniature Schnauzers) and presents with peracute signs of haemorrhagic vomiting and diarrhoea. It may be a clostridial enterotoxaemia and is characterized by a massive outpouring of extracellular fluid (ECF) into the gut, resulting in severe hypovolaemic shock before signs of intracellular dehydration (e.g. altered skin turgor) are seen. A marked increase in the PCV is characteristic, reflecting loss of ECF fluid in excess of the loss of RBCs. Other haematological and biochemical parameters are largely unremarkable, and any abnormalities are the result of hypovolaemia. Hyponatraemia and hyperkalaemia would alert one to the differential diagnosis of hypoadrenocorticism.

ii. The aim of treatment is replacement of fluid loss with aggressive intravenous fluid therapy at initial flow rates up to 90 ml/kg for the first hour. Reduce the flow rate once the PCV falls below 0.55 l/l to a rate necessary to keep the haematocrit at this level. A balanced electrolyte solution is preferred but any isotonic fluid is better than none; fluids are given for 1–3 days depending on the initial severity of the illness and the patient's progress. Some dogs become hypoproteinaemic following aggressive crystalloid fluid therapy; plasma transfusion may be necessary. No other specific therapies have been shown to be beneficial. Prophylactic broad-spectrum bactericidal antibiotics are given as the ulcerated intestine may act as a portal for bacterial entry. Clavulanate-potentiated amoxycillin is usually adequate but some animals may require intravenous cephalosporins, aminoglycosides or metronidazole. The use of corticosteroids is controversial; high doses (1–2 mg/kg i/v) of hydrocortisone or soluble dexamethasone may help in shock, but there is no indication for maintenance doses.

iii. Without treatment the mortality rate is high, but with appropriate therapy the high morbidity is not associated with significant mortality. Death results from hypovolaemic shock, possibly complicated by secondary endotoxaemia and hypoproteinaemia. The recurrence rate is quite high, especially in the toy breeds.

30 i. Hyperthyroidism (thyrotoxicosis).

ii. The commonest cause is benign adenomatous hyperplasia of one or both thyroid lobes resulting in thyroid enlargement (goitre) which can usually be palpated between the larynx and the manubrium.

iii. High basal serum total thyroid hormone concentrations are the biochemical hallmark of hyperthyroidism. In this case the serum total T4 concentration is diagnostically elevated. The corresponding serum total T3 concentration is within the reference range but this does not preclude a diagnosis of hyperthyroidism and occurs in approximately 25% of affected cases. This phenomenon is usually seen in mildly affected cats and it is likely that T3 would increase into the diagnostic range if the disorder was allowed to progress untreated. T3 is secreted by the thyroid gland but up to 60% of circulating T3 is produced peripherally from monodeiodination of T4. Since T3 is more metabolically active than T4, it is possible that autoregulation of this step plays a role in maintaining serum total T3 concentrations within the reference range in the early stages of the disease.

iv. Excess circulating thyroid hormones cause a variety of clinical signs, the commonest of which are weight loss despite a normal or increased appetite, polyuria/polydipsia, hyperactivity and intermittent GI signs of vomiting and/or diarrhoea. Cardiac abnormalities such as tachycardia and murmurs are also common.

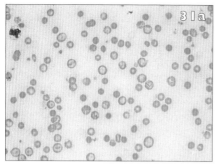 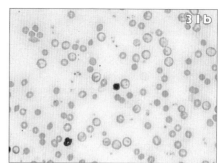

31 A four-year-old, female Collie presents with sudden onset weakness, collapse, pallor and tachycardia four weeks after a season. There are no other significant physical findings except mild pyrexia. An in-house PCV is 0.17 l/l and you elect for a full haematological profile. The profile yields the results shown. Photomicrographs of the blood films are shown (**31a, 31b**).

i. What would your film comment be? Note the morphology of the anaemia.

ii. What type of anaemia is this?

iii. What is the significance of the WBC count?

iv. What is the significance of the nRBCs?

v. What other tests are now indicated?

RBCs ($\times 10^{12}$/l)	1.75
Hb (g/l)	50
PCV (l/l)	0.17
MCV (fl)	98
MCHC (g/l)	290
nRBCs	10%
Platelets ($\times 10^9$/l)	367
WBCs ($\times 10^9$/l)	36.9
Neutrophils (seg) ($\times 10^9$/l)	25.8
Neutrophils (bands) ($\times 10^9$/l)	0.66
Lymphocytes ($\times 10^9$/l)	2.9
Monocytes ($\times 10^9$/l)	0.01
Eosinophils ($\times 10^9$/l)	0.33

32 A two-year-old, male Old English Sheepdog presented with a two-month history of gross haematuria which had been proven on multiple urinalyses. Bacteriology produced no growth on several occasions. Urination was normal but the severity of bleeding varied on a day-to-day basis. As far as the owner was concerned the dog was otherwise well.

i. How would you investigate this dog?

ii. If no gross lesions were found, how would you proceed?

31 i. Corrected WBC count 33.1×10^9/l; nRBCs at various stages; polychromasia +; anisocytosis +; occasional spherocytes; platelet count appears adequate. The WBC count is normally corrected if nRBCs are greater than 10%, because counters using the Coulter principle will count nRBCs as WBCs. The formula for correcting the WBC count is:
corrected WBC count = [100/(100 + nRBCs)] × automated cell count.
ii. This is a macrocytic, hypochromic regenerative anaemia with spherocytosis, typical of autoimmune haemolytic anaemia (AIHA).
iii. There is a neutrophilia with a left shift. This is nearly always present in cases of AIHA and is often assumed to be a reflection of an inflammatory response accompanying AIHA or due to non-specific bone marrow stimulation and possibly damage to the bone marrow sinusoids, resulting in the increased release of granulocytes from the marrow. In this case it could also be due to a concurrent pyometra.
iv. Nucleated RBCs at different stages are present. This is not just due to regeneration. The release of rubricytes as well as metarubricytes implies that there is bone marrow damage/dysfunction present. This is frequently present in cases of AIHA where a leuco-erythroblastic response may be seen, i.e. release of very early RBC and WBC precursors into the circulation.
v. A Coombs test. The direct Coombs test in this case was positive at 1/256.

32 i. • Routine haematology and biochemistry should be performed to assess the level of anaemia, the presence of a regenerative response and for evidence of underlying disease.
• Urine should be collected by cystocentesis and submitted for analysis and bacteriology.
• Ultrasound examination of the kidneys, bladder and prostate to check for anatomical abnormalities/textural change.
• Radiographic examination, consisting of plain abdominal films, an intravenous urogram (IVU), retrograde positive contrast urethrocystogram and double contrast cystogram, allows examination of the whole urinary tract and is complementary to ultrasound examination. Mild irregularity of the kidneys is frequently more obvious on an IVU than ultrasound examination. Vermiform filling deficits suggestive of renal haemorrhage may be seen on an IVU and this technique also allows more thorough evaluation of the ureters.
ii. No abnormalities were found on any of the investigations performed other than gross haematuria on a urine sample obtained by cystocentesis. The signs are consistent with bleeding from the bladder or upper urinary tract. The young age of the dog and the history are suggestive of idiopathic renal haemorrhage. The site of the haemorrhage may be confirmed by catheterizing both ureters via a cystotomy during a period of gross haematuria. In this case there was obvious haematuria from the left ureter whilst urine from the right ureter was grossly normal. The haemorrhage is controlled by performing a ureteronephrectomy on the affected side. The excised kidney and ureter should undergo pathological examination to check for the presence of lesions not detected during radiographic and ultrasonographic investigations. Typically no lesions to account for the blood loss are found in idiopathic renal haemorrhage. Other possible causes of renal haemorrhage: trauma; bleeding diseases; and neoplasia which may be benign (e.g. renal haemangioma) or malignant (e.g. renal carcinoma).

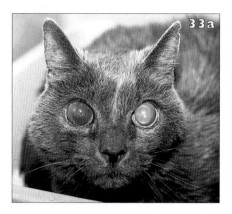
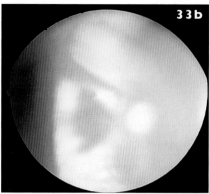

33 A 16-year-old, neutered female domestic shorthair cat is presented for evaluation of acute blindness. The cat has not been eating well and seems to be drinking more water than usual. Physical examination reveals a thin cat with pale mucous membranes. There is no menace response but other cranial nerve responses appear to be intact. The pupils are dilated and do not respond to light (**33a**). A fundic examination is performed (**33b**).
i. What is your diagnosis?
ii. List three ways that systemic blood pressure can be measured.
iii. In addition to ocular changes, name three other organ systems that may be affected by systemic hypertension.
iv. Name three systemic diseases that may be associated with systemic hypertension.
v. List three classes of drugs used to treat systemic hypertension. Give an example of each and their mechanism of action.

34 This radiograph (**34**) is of a dog which presented with acute (few hours duration) persistent retching and vomiting and severe depression of several hours' duration. The dog was inappetent but attempted to drink. Hypersalivation was present.
i. What is your diagnosis?
ii. How would you treat this case?
iii. How would you feed this dog once its problem had been resolved?

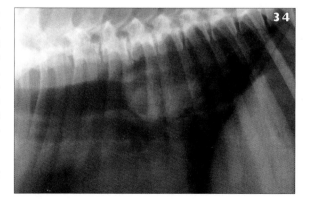

33 i. Retinal vessels tortuosity, haemorrhage and detachment.

ii. Systemic arterial blood pressure may be measured directly by cannulating an artery or indirectly using Doppler ultrasound or oscillometry.

iii. Cardiovascular system – left ventricular hypertrophy, vascular hypertrophy; brain – haemorrhage; kidneys – renal failure.

iv. Chronic renal failure, hyperthyroidism, hyperadrenocorticism, phaeochromocytoma.

v. Antihypertensive agents are shown below:

Drug class	Mechanism of action	Example(s)
Angiotensin converting enzyme (ACE) inhibitor	Impairs ACE activity resulting in decreased angiotensin II production	enalapril captopril lisinopril
Calcium channel blocking agent	Smooth muscle relaxation	diltiazem amlodipine verapamil
Diuretic	a. Inhibits sodium chloride transport in loop of Henle b. Blocks aldosterone receptor c. Distal nephron diuretic	a. frusemide (furosemide) b. spironolactone c. chlorothiazide, hydrochlorothiazide
Arterial vasodilator	Direct arteriolar dilator	hydralazine nitroprusside
Beta-adrenergic antagonists	Decreased cardiac output, heart rate and sympathetic tone	propranolol atenolol labetalol
Alpha-adrenergic antagonist	Peripheral arteriolar vasodilation	prazosin

34 i. The radiograph shows a large mineral density within the oesophagus, consistent with a bony oesophageal foreign body.

ii. Removal of most oesophageal foreign bodies can be achieved through the mouth (endoscopically or fluoroscopically). If this fails, removal through a gastrostomy can be attempted. Removal through a thoracotomy is the least preferable method as oesophageal healing is poor. Oesophageal mucosal damage invariably develops. Oesophagitis is painful and thus analgesics such as a narcotic analgesic or a NSAID are indicated postoperatively. The use of anti-inflammatory doses of prednisolone may reduce stricture formation. Gastro-oesophageal reflux may occur and thus the use of an H_2-blocker (cimetidine, ranitidine) may be helpful. Prophylactic antibacterial therapy is indicated.

iii. Nil by mouth is recommended for 7–10 days to allow the oesophagus to heal and to reduce the risk of stricture formation. Placement of a gastrostomy feeding tube endoscopically at the time of the initial anaesthetic is indicated.

35 A young male dog presented with dysuria and haematuria of several days' duration. The prostate was painful and a prostatic wash contained numerous degenerate and non-degenerate neutrophils, and gram-negative rods. Radiographically, the prostate was enlarged. At exploratory laparotomy a prostatic abscess was found (35).

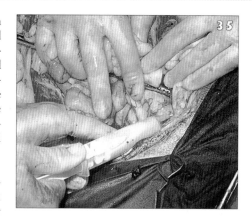

i. How would you treat this case?
ii. If this was a case of chronic prostatitis, what considerations would you take into account when planning your antibacterial treatment?

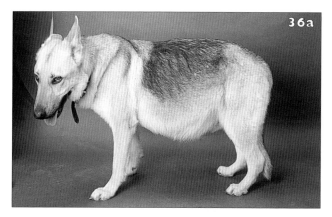

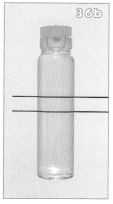

36 A six-year-old, male German Shepherd Dog presents with diarrhoea and abdominal enlargement (36a). A fluid wave is detected by ballottement and clear fluid is obtained by abdominocentesis. The fluid is a transudate (36b) and serum biochemistry confirms hypoalbuminaemia (13 g/l).
i. What are the characteristics of a transudate?
ii. What are the major disease processes causing hypoalbuminaemia?
iii. Briefly describe how would you distinguish between the causes of hypoalbuminaemia.

35 i. The prostatic abscess should be drained. This can be achieved by either marsupializing the prostate to the ventral body wall or by placing a drain through the body wall into the prostate. In this case a Foley catheter was placed into the prostatic abscess and held in place by inflating the bulb with water. This allowed the abscess to be drained twice daily for seven days. Enrofloxacin was administered for four weeks as the organism isolated was a resistant *E. coli*. The dog was also castrated in order to reduce prostatic size and to limit the possibility of chronic prostatitis developing.

ii. Acute prostatitis or prostatic abscesses may be treated with a wide range of antibacterials as the blood-prostate barrier is not usually intact in acute inflammation. However, with chronic prostatitis antibiotic penetration and activity in the prostate is limited by the acidic environment of the prostatic acini compared with the interstitium. Therefore, basic antibiotics such as erythromycin, clindamycin and trimethoprim become trapped in the acini resulting in high concentrations of these antibiotics. Lipid soluble drugs, such as chloramphenicol, trimethoprim, macrolides and fluoroquinolones, also enter the acini in high concentrations. The usual sulphonamide components in trimethoprim-sulphonamide combinations do not enter the prostate well. Thus, when treating chronic prostatitis, or as a follow-on antibiotic after treatment of acute prostatitis, one of the antibiotics listed above should be used. Castration is also recommended.

36 i. A transudate is clear and characteristically has a specific gravity of <1.017, a total protein of <25 g/l and <1,000 cells per μl.

ii. Starvation and chronic inflammatory diseases can cause mild hypoalbuminaemia, although this is never sufficient to cause an ascitic transudate. The three major classes of disease causing hypoalbuminaemia are: protein-losing nephropathy (PLN); liver failure; protein-losing enteropathy (PLE).

iii. Crude separation of hepatic, renal and intestinal causes of hypoalbuminaemia can be made by comparing the serum globulin concentrations. In general, globulin is increased in liver disease, normal in PLNs and decreased in PLEs. Clinical signs are often helpful, as chronic diarrhoea would be expected in a PLE. PLN is easily diagnosed by looking for proteinuria, with the urine protein:creatinine ratio being the most reliable index in practice. Liver failure is assessed by bile acid concentrations. A PLE can only be confirmed by measuring faecal loss of [51]chromium radio-labelled albumin, but this test is not applicable to practice. Measurement of the faecal excretion of an endogenous protein resistant to digestion, such as α–1 protease inhibitor, may be a useful test. Currently, after hepatic and renal disease has been ruled out, a diagnosis of a PLE is pursued by intestinal biopsy.

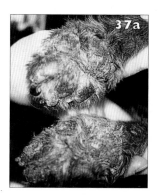

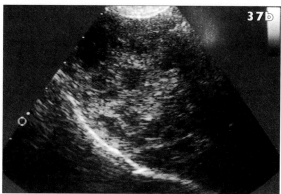

37 A ten-year-old, entire male Cocker Spaniel presented for evaluation of a progressive, suppurative paronychia of all four feet (37a). Soaking the feet in drying agents decreased the exudation but long-term antibiotic therapy had not elicited an improvement. The foot pads were crusted and cracked and the nail beds were deformed. Crusting, ulcerative lesions on the oral mucocutaneous junctions and scrotum, and hyperkeratosis of the nasal planum were present. Results of initial blood work are shown.

i. What are the differential diagnoses for the skin lesions?

ii. Could there be a connection between the skin lesions and the biochemical and ultrasonographic abnormalities (37b)?

iii. What further diagnostic tests are indicated?

iv. What are the treatment options and prognosis?

PCV (l/l)	0.33
WBCs ($\times 10^9$/l)	16.2
Neutrophils - segmented ($\times 10^9$/l)	14.9
Lymphocytes ($\times 10^9$/l)	0.8
Monocytes ($\times 10^9$/l)	0.5
Platelets ($\times 10^9$/l)	262
Urine SG	1.047
Albumin (g/l)	21
Globulin (g/l)	38
Bilirubin (µmol/l)	5.7
ALT (u/l)	470
ALP (u/l)	2,738
Cholesterol (mmol/l)	10.8
Bile acids – fasted (µmol/l)	42
Bile acids – postprandial (µmol/l)	89
Glucose (mmol/l)	7.6

38 Your client is a cat rescuer. Euthanasia of a sick FIV-positive queen had been performed recently. Now she brings in the queen's three eight-week-old kittens to be tested for FIV antibodies.

i. Are you going to perform the test?

ii. If not, why not?

iii. If so, what advice will you give?

37 & 38: Answers

37 i. The erosive crusting of the nasal planum, oral mucocutaneous junctions, foot pads and genitalia can occur in diseases such as pemphigus foliaceus, drug eruption, lupus erythematosus, necrolytic migratory erythema, zinc-responsive dermatosis and generic dog food dermatoses.

ii. The skin lesions, in conjunction with the abnormal liver parameters, are suggestive of a diagnosis of necrolytic migratory erythema or so-called hepatocutaneous syndrome. The ultrasound of the liver demonstrates the patchy appearance of hypoechoic nodules within a hyperechoic background which is characteristic of this disease.

iii. The diagnosis of hepatocutaneous syndrome is strongly suspected based on the clinical findings so far. A definitive diagnosis may be made with characteristic skin and liver histopathology demonstrating hyperkeratosis and intracellular oedema and periportal vacuolar hepatopathy, respectively. In humans this syndrome is most often associated with a glucagon-secreting pancreatic tumour. In dogs, glucagonomas have been identified but are very rare.

iv. A majority of affected dogs have been found to have severe reductions in plasma amino acid concentrations, and the addition of high-protein sources such as egg yolk to the diet has produced considerable improvement in some dogs. Prednisolone has also been shown to improve the cutaneous lesions in some dogs, but approximately 90% of these dogs have abnormal glucose tolerance and hyperglucagonaemia, and the insulin antagonistic effects of steroids may contribute to the development of fulminant diabetes mellitus. Unfortunately, the prognosis of affected dogs is poor to guarded.

38 i. No.

ii. Eight-week-old kittens of an FIV-positive cat are likely to test FIV antibody positive because they usually still have circulating maternally derived antibodies. No true assessment of whether or not they are infected can be made at this stage. Wait until they are 16 weeks of age or older and then test them. Since FIV is infrequently transmitted from queen to kitten, it is very likely that the kittens will test negative at this stage. If for some reason their FIV infection status has to be known immediately, then you would need to find a laboratory which routinely detects the virus itself, usually by culture of WBCs or by PCR testing as it becomes more widely available.

iii. If you test the kittens now, they will probably be positive and you would advise that they be retested after 16 weeks of age for the reasons given in **ii.** above. For most cat rescuers money is short and two tests would be wasteful.

39 A fourteen-week-old, male Boxer puppy presented with a two-week history of incoordination, initially in the hindlimbs but eventually involving the forelimbs, which had progressed to paralysis. There was no history of vomiting or diarrhoea, exposure to toxins or rubbish eating and the dog had only been allowed access to the owner's garden. Two days prior to referral the pup

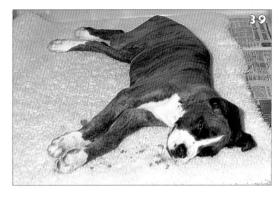

developed dysphagia. On presentation the pup was recumbent (39) but bright and alert. He was unable to stand due to a flaccid paralysis affecting all four limbs. No voluntary movement of the limbs was possible and no spinal reflexes (e.g. patella, withdrawal or panniculus reflexes) could be elicited. All conscious proprioceptive reflexes were absent. Marked abdominal breathing was evident and the gag reflex was reduced. All other cranial nerves appeared unaffected. The pup was faecally and urinary continent and was able to feel pain. The rectal temperature was unremarkable and cardiovascular criteria were within normal limits.

i. What diagnoses would you consider?
ii. What diagnostic tests would you recommend?
iii. How would you treat your most likely diagnosis?

40 You perform a postmortem examination on a four-week-old faded kitten. Your veterinary laboratory diagnoses feline herpes virus 1 (FHV-1, also called feline rhinotracheitis virus) as the likely cause of fading.
i. In which two ways might you have sent the lung samples from the kitten for the laboratory to reach this diagnosis?
ii. Your assistant suggests that you take an oropharyngeal swab into viral transport medium from the queen to see if she is a carrier. Is this a good idea? Would you expect her to be shedding FHV-1?
iii. If the queen is a carrier of FHV-1, will she ever be free of infection?
iv. Would vaccination help to eliminate the virus?
v. Can the queen be used again for breeding?

39 i. The neurological abnormalities (i.e. generalized paralysis with loss of reflexes) are consistent with a lower motor neuron disorder. The disease process may be affecting the peripheral nerves, the neuromuscular junction or the nerve cell bodies in the ventral grey matter of the spinal cord. Hindlimbs are often affected more severely at first, although forelimbs usually become involved with many degenerative or inflammatory neuropathies. The main differential diagnosis for lower motor neuron disorders in a dog of this age is an inflammatory infectious disorder (e.g. toxoplasmosis, neosporosis). Other conditions which may result in similar signs were thought less likely given the acute onset and the age of the dog. These included:
• Congenital and familial disorders of demyelination and axonal degeneration. They would normally present in older animals with a longer clinical course and with other neurological deficits.
• Polyneuropathies associated with metabolic, toxic or neoplastic disease. No history of ingestion of toxins.
• Neuromuscular junction disorders, e.g. botulism, tick paralysis. No exposure to dead animals or ticks.
• Inflammatory immune-mediated disorders of the central/peripheral nervous system. Too young.
ii. Clinical biochemistry and haematological assessment are indicated. Serology for toxoplasmosis and neosporosis is required. CSF analysis is indicated to assess for an inflammatory disorder. Electromyography can also be carried out as a protozoal myositis may accompany an encephalitis.
iii. Treatment of a protozoal encephalitis is unrewarding. Clindamycin or trimethoprim/sulphonamide with pyrimethamine may be helpful. Euthanasia is often required because of respiratory paralysis before any treatment has had a chance to be effective. Nutritional support is required where treatment is attempted. Placement of a nasogastric tube would allow for provision of food and water.

40 i. In virus transport medium for virus isolation, or in formalin for histopathology. In FHV-1 infection there are intranuclear inclusion bodies.
ii. FHV-1 is shed from the oropharynx after a stressful event for up to three weeks. It is likely that by four weeks after parturition, FHV-1 shedding has ceased, therefore a negative finding would not rule out FHV-1 infection. A positive swab would show the queen to be a FHV-1 carrier. Examination of the history would be useful. If the queen was isolated with her kittens from birth, then the kittens can only have been infected by the queen, indirect transmission via the owner being unlikely.
iii. No. Latent FHV-1 infection is lifelong; it is believed that latent FHV-1 inhabits the trigeminal nerve ganglia.
iv. Vaccination makes no difference to an already infected cat.
v. It is probably not a good idea to breed from a queen which repeatedly produces FHV-1 infected litters; FHV-1 can infect kittens as they are born. However, if the breeder is determined to try, boost the cat with vaccine before conception so that levels of maternally derived antibody are high. Wean the kittens at 2–3 weeks of age, isolate them from their mother and vaccinate intranasally every three weeks until they are old enough for a parenteral vaccine at 8–9 weeks of age.

Analysis	Pre-treatment	Post-treatment
Urea (mmol/l)	9.0	38.0
Creatinine (µmol/l)	119	320
Phosphate (mmol/l)	3.40	8.16
Total T4 (nmol/l)	455	30

41 The above biochemical abnormalities were obtained from a 14-year-old cat both before and one week after commencing carbimazole therapy for hyperthyroidism (5 mg q8h).
i. What is your interpretation of these results?
ii. Would these results be seen with other therapeutic protocols for hyperthyroidism?

42 A seven and a half-year-old, entire male Cocker Spaniel was presented with haematuria of several months' duration. The blood was always mixed with urine and tended to be worst towards the end of urination. Radiographic and ultrasonographic investigations revealed the lesions shown (**42a, 42b**).
i. What is your main differential diagnosis?
ii. How would you treat this animal, and what complications may occur?

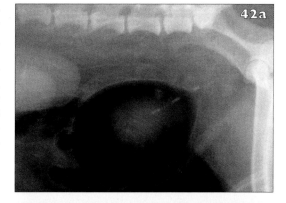

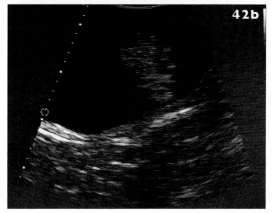

41 i. Treatment-induced renal dysfunction. Prior to treatment the serum total thyroxine concentration is markedly elevated and confirms the diagnosis of hyperthyroidism. The serum urea and creatinine concentrations are within the reference range; mild hyperphosphataemia has been described in hyperthyroid cats without evidence of renal disease. The results following treatment indicate successful induction of euthyroidism but with a severe deterioration of renal function. An increase in serum urea and creatinine concentrations with the development, in some cases, of overt renal disease has been associated with treatment of hyperthyroidism. This is presumably related to a decrease in the glomerular filtration rate allowing emergence of pre-existing renal disease.

ii. This is not a specific effect of carbimazole therapy but rather the reversal of the hyperthyroid state; similar results are found in cats treated with radioactive iodine or by surgical thyroidectomy.

42 i. The main differential diagnosis is polypoid cystitis; this is based upon the size, position and number of the intravesicular masses. On ultrasound examination of the bladder the polyps do not invade the bladder wall but appear to arise from the urothelium. However, the diagnosis should be confirmed histopathologically.

ii. Any underlying cause for the polypoid cystitis should be sought and treated, e.g. calculi, urinary tract infection. Polypoid cystitis is a poorly defined condition but is thought to occur secondary to chronic bladder irritation. Animals may show signs of haematuria and occasionally urinary frequency, but may also be asymptomatic. Treatment may be medical or surgical. In some cases the polyps may resolve spontaneously following treatment of a urinary tract infection or dissolution of urinary calculi. However, in persistent cases or where cystic calculi require removal the diagnosis is usually confirmed and the animal treated concomitantly by performing excisional biopsies of the masses. A ventral cystotomy allows good access to the bladder lumen. The bladder is everted and each polyp isolated by applying some mosquito forceps at the base of the polyp. The polyp is excised and the forceps left in place for several minutes until haemostasis is achieved. This technique absolves the use of suture material within the bladder lumen. The main complication of the surgery is haemorrhage. This is usually minor and self-limiting; however, if severe haemorrhage occurs during recovery, a clot may form within the bladder lumen. This may obstruct the bladder neck, like a ball valve, causing postoperative obstruction or dysuria. The risk of this occurring may be reduced by encouraging frequent urination and creating a diuresis by administering intravenous fluids.

43 A ten-year-old, female Labrador Retriever presents with a history of weight gain, exercise intolerance and two episodes of collapse in the past two and a half weeks. Her abdomen is very tense and the caudal edges of the liver are not palpably distinguishable from the surrounding viscera. Pertinent biochemical abnormalities include increased serum liver enzyme activities (ALT

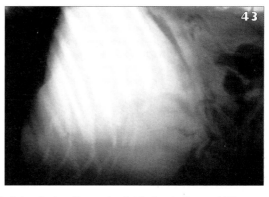

2,849 u/l, ALP 2,959 u/l). A lateral abdominal radiograph of this dog is shown (43).
i. Describe the radiographic abnormalities.
ii. Discuss a list of differential diagnoses.
iii. What further diagnostic tests might be indicated?

44 Your client has five cats ranging from 2–12 years of age. All the cats are fully vaccinated and boosted against FeLV infection. He wants to introduce a pedigree kitten, but the breeder will not let him have the kitten until he has his existing cats tested for FeLV. Your client points out that his cats have been FeLV vaccinated and that he intends to vaccinate the kitten too. He comes to you for advice: should he test all his cats or not?

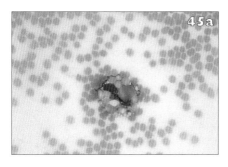
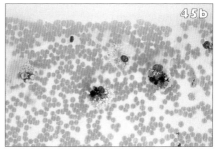

45 Two photomicrographs of cytology preparations made by centrifugation of a pericardial effusion are shown (45a, 45b). They are stained with Wright's stain.
i. What is the structure in the centre of 45a?
ii. Which features of the cells in these photomicrographs indicate the presence of old/past haemorrhage?

43 i. The caudal border of the liver is indistinct and extends beyond the costochondral junction. The stomach and loops of small intestine are displaced caudally and dorsally indicating a massive hepatomegaly.

ii. The severity of the hepatic enlargement in this dog is more likely the result of a liver mass, cyst, abscess or other such space occupying disease.

iii. An ultrasound examination of the liver is useful to define the inner architecture of the organ and differentiate between the presence of a solid mass and a hypoechogenic cyst or abscess. Ultrasound can also help to direct a needle or biopsy instrument to the affected area to obtain a tissue sample for cytological and/or histopathological analysis. This dog had a large, solid mass consuming the middle liver lobe.

44 Yes. All the cats should be tested as any of them could be excreting FeLV. No FeLV vaccine is 100% effective and vaccination is not a substitute for testing in the prevention of FeLV. The only circumstance in which your client would not need to test would be if the cats had all been tested twice, at a 12 week interval, before vaccination and had been kept in a closed environment ever since (i.e. with no access to outdoors and other cats). If all cats test FeLV negative at the same time, it is likely that the household is FeLV free (since in a household where FeLV is endemic, 40% of cats are usually infected). If some test negative and others positive, the cats should be retested as the negative cats may be in the early stages of infection and not yet viraemic (the incubation period from infection to viraemia is around 21 days). To avoid retesting after 12 weeks test the negative cats for virus neutralizing antibodies (VNA). If a good titre is present (≥32), then the cats are immune and there is no need to retest them; it will be safe to mix them with positive cats. If a cat's VNA titre is zero, then an antigen retest will still be necessary for that cat. The kitten itself should be tested unless the breeder can produce evidence that every cat in the cattery has been FeLV tested negative within the previous year.

45 i. A macrophage distended with phagocytosed RBCs.

ii. There are no platelet clumps among the RBCs to indicate fresh haemorrhage. The macrophages present here exhibit erythrophagocytosis and also contain blood breakdown pigments (dark green/black and orange), and one macrophage in **45b** contains a bright orange haematoidin crystal.

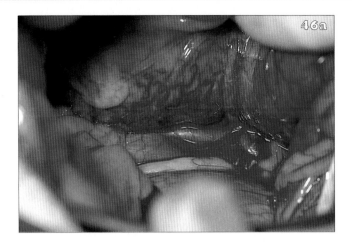

46 A two-year-old, male German Shepherd Dog developed abdominal enlargement over four weeks and became inappetent. Abdominal radiography showed marked loss of detail due to abdominal effusion. Abdominocentesis yielded serosanguinous fluid (protein 27 g/l, nucleated cell count 1.2 × 10⁹/l). Laboratory analysis revealed mild elevation of liver enzymes (ALT 228 u/l, ALP 318 u/l). Exploratory laparotomy revealed many tortuous vessels in the mesocolon and around the left kidney (46a). The liver looked slightly irregular.

i. What are your differential diagnoses for the ascites?
ii. What other tests could you have done before surgery to further define the problem?
iii. What are the vessels seen during surgery?

47 This 12-year-old, neutered female cat presented with a plantigrade posture and a prolonged history of polyuria/polydipsia (47).

i. What is the most likely diagnosis?
ii. How would you confirm the diagnosis?

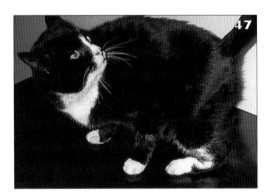

46 i. The main presenting problem in this dog is ascites which may be classified as a transudate, modified transudate or exudate, based on peritoneal fluid analysis. The fluid in this dog was a modified transudate, which may be caused by liver disease, portal hypertension, congestive heart failure (unlikely in this case), posthepatic venous obstruction (e.g. vena caval disease) or neoplasia.

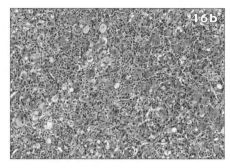

ii. Cytological examination of the ascitic fluid would have been helpful to look for the presence of neoplastic cells. Serum bile acid determination should have been performed in order to investigate for possible liver dysfunction. Abdominal ultrasound could have allowed for better examination of the abdomen and would have been particularly useful to assess liver size, hepatic parenchyma and biliary system. If bile acid determination and/or hepatic ultrasonography had indicated liver disease, a percutaneous ultrasound-guided liver biopsy could have been taken; this is less invasive than a laparotomy.

iii. The vessels seen at surgery are multiple extrahepatic portosystemic shunts, which develop as a result of chronic, severe liver disease and portal hypertension. They are frequently seen around the left kidney, as in this case. This is an indication to biopsy the liver. Liver biopsy (H&E stain) in this dog showed diffuse pericellular hepatic fibrosis and distortion of the lobule (46b). Idiopathic hepatic fibrosis has been reported in young dogs (German Shepherd Dogs are predisposed) with evidence of chronic hepatic failure, portal hypertension and hepatic encephalopathy. Symptomatic treatment has resulted in long-term survival in a number of dogs, although generally the prognosis is guarded.

47 i. Diabetes mellitus. The plantigrade posture where the cat walks with its hocks touching the ground is a not uncommon presenting feature of diabetes mellitus in the cat and presumably results from a peripheral neuropathy. Such a diagnosis is supported by the history of polyuria/polydipsia.

ii. By demonstrating a fasting hyperglycaemia and glucosuria. Persistence of these findings on serial sampling is important to eliminate other possible causes of glucosuria and hyperglycaemia, particularly stress-induced hyperglycaemia which commonly occurs in cats. If ketones are also present in the urine, a diagnosis of diabetes mellitus is confirmed. Other non-specific but supportive abnormalities include hypercholesterolaemia, increased activities of alanine aminotransferase (ALT) and alkaline phosphatase (ALP), hyperbilirubinaemia and a stress leucogram with a mild non-regenerative anaemia.

48 A young crossbreed dog has irregular cavities in its permanent dentition when the teeth emerge (48). Prior history is of acute diarrhoea as a puppy.
i. What is the lesion, and what is its cause?
ii. What clinical significance does it hold?

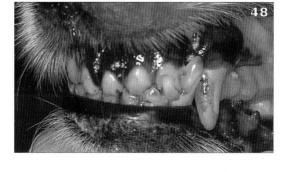

49 This kidney (49) is from a dog which presented with a two-week history of polyuria/polydipsia. Two days prior to presentation the dog had become depressed and anorectic and had vomited. He had not been observed to urinate in the preceding 12 hours. The peripheral lymph nodes and liver were enlarged, and cranial abdominal pain was recorded. Clinical biochemistry was performed; the abnormal results are shown.
i. What diagnoses would you consider in this case?
ii. What treatment options are available to you to manage hypercalcaemia?

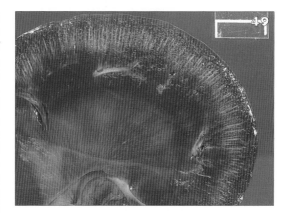

ALT (u/l)	230
ALP (u/l)	790
Bile acids (µmol/l)	23
Urea (mmol/l)	65
Creatinine (µmol/l)	1,240
Calcium (mmol/l)	4.9
Phosphate (mmol/l)	1.4

50 A six-month-old, male Toy Poodle has one testicle present within the scrotum. The other testicle is not palpable.
i. What is the likely condition from which this dog is suffering?
ii. What treatment options are available?
iii. Is this abnormality inherited, and what advice should be given to the breeder?

48 i. Enamel hypoplasia. In light of the earlier history it is consistent with previous distemper infection.

ii. Although having no significance at this time, except as a cosmetic defect, if chorea or seizures develop in later life, distemper as a cause of 'old-dog encephalitis' must be considered.

49 i. The biochemistry is consistent with severe renal failure. Assessment of urine SG would have been helpful in distinguishing between acute (oliguric) and chronic (polyuric) renal failure. However, the acute onset of the signs, the absence of any previous signs of polyuria and polydipsia, and the presence of a severe hypercalcaemia would suggest that this was more likely to be acute renal failure secondary to hypercalcaemia. The gross appearance of the kidney is consistent with hypercalcaemic nephropathy; calcinosis of the tubules is evident. The coexistence of hypercalcaemia and a peripheral lymphadenopathy are strongly suggestive of lymphoma. The vomiting is most likely to be secondary to the renal failure.

ii. Fluid therapy (0.9% saline) and frusemide should be administered to manage the acute renal failure and to promote calcium excretion. An initial flow rate of up to 100 ml/kg/hr may be required, but beware of overhydration by weighing the patient regularly and monitoring respiratory function and urine output. After a couple of hours the flow rate should be reduced to 150 ml/kg/day. If hypercalcaemia persists, calcium lowering drugs such as salcatonin, clodronate, etidronate or pamidronate may be prescribed. None of these are veterinary licensed products in the UK. The use of prednisolone as a means of lowering calcium levels should be avoided as it may induce resistance to cytotoxic drugs which may be used in the management of lymphoma.

50 i. Cryptorchidism (hidden testicle). The testicle may be intra-abdominal, inguinal or ectopic (present in the femoral triangle, caudal perineum or cranial to the scrotum). Cryptorchidism may be unilateral or bilateral. The term monorchidism (single testicle in the body) is often wrongly used since this condition is extremely rare and most cases are unilateral cryptorchids with a single abdominal testicle. The testes normally descend into the scrotum following contraction of the gubernaculum testis by ten days after birth; however, a diagnosis of cryptorchidism is not usually made until after 12 weeks of age. Cases of delayed testicular descent are probably part of the cryptorchid syndrome.

ii. Various combinations of gonadotrophins and reproductive steroids have been shown to be ineffective in causing testicular descent. Regardless of their lack of effect, these treatments are not ethical considering the likely inherited nature of the condition. The non-scrotal testis has a high risk of neoplasia, therefore it should be removed. Removal of the scrotal testis is necessary to prevent breeding since these dogs are usually fertile.

iii. Cryptorchidism is likely to have a genetic base, and although the mode of inheritance is not known for all breeds, it follows the model of a sex-limited autosomal recessive trait. This means that both female and male parents carry the gene whilst only homozygous males will be cryptorchid. The affected dog should be removed from the breeding programme, as should both parents, since whilst appearing phenotypically normal, they are heterozygous carriers and will transmit the gene to half of their offspring.

51 A three-year-old bitch commenced proestrus 11 days previously. She escaped from her owner and returned six hours later. A vaginal smear has been obtained and stained with a modified Wright-Giemsa stain (51).

i. Has a mating occurred, and if so, is it likely to have been fertile?

ii. How reliably can mating be confirmed in the bitch?

iii. What treatment options are there for an unwanted mating?

52 A two-year-old, neutered female Basset Hound is presented with a history of several weeks' intermittent lethargy, anorexia and slight increase in thirst. More recently the dog has been vomiting and has now developed haemorrhagic diarrhoea. The laboratory results shown were obtained.

i. How would you interpret these laboratory results?

ii. How would you confirm your tentative diagnosis?

RBCs ($\times 10^{12}$/l)	5.5
PCV (l/l)	0.39
Hb (g/l)	139
Platelets ($\times 10^9$/l)	289
WBCs ($\times 10^9$/l)	11.3
White cell differential	Unremarkable
Albumin (g/l)	35
Globulin (g/l)	33
Sodium (mmol/l)	128
Potassium (mmol/l)	7.9
Calcium (mmol/l)	2.9
Urea (mmol/l)	23
Creatinine (µmol/l)	256
ALT (u/l)	43
ALP (u/l)	51
Urine SG	1.025

53 A four-year-old, unilateral cryptorchid male dog is presented with bilaterally symmetric non-pruritic alopecia, gynaecomastia and attractiveness to male dogs. You suspect hyperoestrogenism secondary to a testicular tumour.

i. What hormone analysis may be helpful in the diagnosis?

ii. What possible haematological complications may develop with this condition?

51–53: Answers

51 i. The smear shows large intermediate epithelial cells, red blood cells and spermatozoa. The bitch is in proestrus, and as dog spermatozoa survive within the reproductive tract of the bitch for seven days after mating, this mating could result in pregnancy.

ii. It can be difficult to confirm a mating unless directly observed. Spermatozoa can be detected using a simple vaginal smear technique for only a short period of time after mating. When matings have occurred more than 24 hours previously, an accurate assessment can only be made by centrifugation of a sample to concentrate any spermatozoa present. Sperm that are present within the vagina often lose their tails.

iii. The simplest option is ovariohysterectomy after the end of oestrus. Alternatively, prevent implantation, or wait until a positive diagnosis of pregnancy has been made before inducing abortion or resorption. Oestradiol benzoate, given at a relatively high dose within 4 days of mating or at a low dose on days 3 and 5 (and possibly also day 7) after mating is efficacious. The use of oestradiol benzoate should be considered carefully as it causes uterine disorders and blood dyscrasias (anaemia and thrombocytopenia). This drug is rarely used in the USA because of these adverse effects. The low-dose regime reduces the possibility of adverse effects. Repeated low doses of the prostaglandin analogue cloprostenol reduces plasma progesterone concentration and induces abortion, especially if given later than 25 days after the luteinizing hormone surge. Prostaglandins commonly produce adverse effects including salivation, vomiting and diarrhoea. Prolactin antagonists (bromocriptine and cabergoline) reduce plasma concentrations of progesterone and induce resorption or abortion. Oral cabergoline and injectable cloprostenol together induce pregnancy termination after day 25. This regime reduces the adverse effects of prostaglandin therapy, increases the efficacy of prolactin antagonists, which alone work best after day 40, and appears to be 100% effective.

52 i. Subtle chronic disease and acute GI signs are suspicious of hypoadrenocorticism; the electrolyte values are suggestive. Azotaemia is most likely pre-renal in origin as hyponatraemia causes hypovolaemia and poor renal perfusion. The urine is somewhat concentrated indicating some renal tubular activity, but it is not fully concentrated because of hyponatraemia. Mild hypercalcaemia may be seen in this disease. This dog may be anaemic, but this will not be recognized until ECF volume is restored.

ii. By the ACTH stimulation test before life-time steroid replacement therapy is started.

53 i. Plasma oestrogen (oestradiol) concentrations may be elevated, although in some cases it may be within the reference range. A normal oestrogen concentration does not preclude a diagnosis in the face of appropriate clinical signs. Serum inhibin concentrations have been found to be elevated in a small number of dogs. However, this assay is not available and has not been fully assessed.

ii. Bone marrow hypoplasia and pancytopenia may develop following exposure to increased oestrogen concentrations. Initially, granulocytopoiesis and a neutrophilic leucocytosis develop. Subsequently, hypoplasia of all cell lines and pancytopenia occurs. This is characterized haematologically by variable degrees of non-regenerative anaemia, lymphocytosis and thrombocytopenia.

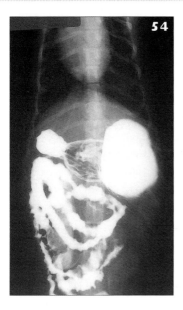

Total protein (g/l)	28
Albumin (g/l)	12
Globulin (g/l)	18
ALT (u/l)	45
ALP (u/l)	300
Urea (mmol/l)	5.6
Creatinine (μmol/l)	68
Glucose (mmol/l)	4.7
Sodium (mmol/l)	150
Potassium (mmol/l)	4.7
Chloride (mmol/l)	120
Calcium (mmol/l)	2.3
Phosphate (mmol/l)	0.9
RBCs ($\times 10^{12}$/l)	4.43
Hb (g/l)	69
PCV (l/l)	0.32
WBCs ($\times 10^9$/l)	4.8
Neutrophils (seg) ($\times 10^9$/l)	3.4
Neutrophils (bands) ($\times 10^9$/l)	0.0
Lymphocytes ($\times 10^9$/l)	1.1
Monocytes ($\times 10^9$/l)	0.2
Eosinophils ($\times 10^9$/l)	0.1

54 A nine-year-old crossbreed dog presented with chronic diarrhoea (watery/pasty) of several months' duration. His appetite had been good but recently he had become inappetent. Polydipsia was not present. The dog had lost 10kg in weight (present weight 20 kg). Subjectively, the walls of the small intestine were thicker than normal. All other abdominal organs, the peripheral lymph nodes, the mucous membranes and thoracic auscultation were unremarkable. Clinical pathology results are shown. The urine protein:creatinine ratio was 0.2. Plain abdominal radiographs were unremarkable. A barium study was performed (**54**).
i. What is your interpretation of the clinical pathology?
ii. What is your interpretation of the radiograph?
iii. How would you proceed with this case?

55 During the investigation of a cat with chronic small intestinal diarrhoea, breath hydrogen excretion is monitored after the administration of xylose (3 g/kg p/o as a 10% aqueous solution). The breath hydrogen profile obtained is shown (**55a**).

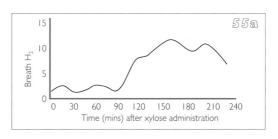

i. What does this test indicate?
ii. What is the basis for this test, and what is its clinical value?

54 i. Diarrhoea with weight loss in spite of a good appetite is consistent with a malabsorptive or maldigestive disorder. The low albumin and globulin are consistent with protein loss, either through the intestinal tract or in the urine; a protein-losing nephropathy (PLN), however, would be highly unlikely with the normal urine protein:creatinine ratio. Haematologically there is a mild normochromic, normocytic anaemia, possibly an anaemia of chronic disease, or it may reflect the protein deficiency.

ii. The radiograph shows multiple filling defects along the entire wall of the small intestinal tract. This is typical of the so-called 'apple core appearance' and is usually associated with alimentary lymphoma or severe inflammatory bowel disease (IBD). No other significant abnormalities are evident.

iii. An intestinal biopsy, obtained endoscopically or at a laparotomy, is required to distinguish between alimentary lymphoma and severe IBD. Both carry very poor prognoses, although IBD is potentially manageable.

55 i. Xylose malassimilation; this indicates the presence of small intestinal disease.

ii. The test works on the principle that the only hydrogen present in exhaled breath is derived from bacterial fermentation of carbohydrates in the large intestine. In a healthy starved animal, xylose (a simple sugar or monosaccharide) (circles in **55b**) given by mouth is completely absorbed in the small intestine so no carbohydrate is available to the colonic bacteria (rods in **55b**); the breath hydrogen concentration remains low (typically 1–2 ppm). In a cat with malassimilation (malabsorption), some of the xylose may pass to the large intestine where bacterial fermentation results in hydrogen production, detected as an increase in breath hydrogen concentration. In this cat, breath hydrogen concentration rises appreciably after about 90 minutes, which would be compatible with the time taken for aqueous xylose to pass to the colon. The test is a simple, non-invasive way of demonstrating malassimilation, which usually indicates an infiltrative small intestinal disease such as inflammatory bowel disease, or a diffuse intestinal lymphoma.

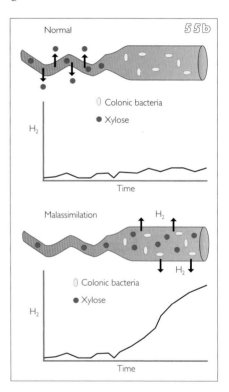

56 This photograph (56) shows the oral mucous membranes of a ten-year-old, neutered female crossbreed dog with anorexia, vomiting and jaundice of three days' duration. Previously she had been in good health. Her vaccinations were current. Two weeks before she became ill she had undergone a routine dental under general anaesthesia and was given trimethoprim/sulphadiazine for three days afterwards.

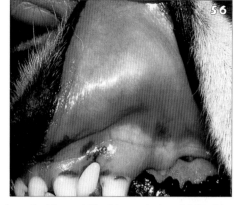

Haematology revealed PCV 0.48 l/l, WBC 27.8 × 10⁹/l and normal platelets. A serum biochemical profile showed marked hyperbilirubinaemia (total bilirubin 648 µmol/l), elevated liver enzymes (ALT 1,224 u/l, ALP 1,058 u/l), hypoglycaemia (3.0 mmol/l) and low-normal cholesterol (2.2 mmol/l). Plain abdominal radiographs were normal.

i. What are your differential diagnoses?
ii. Would liver biopsy be indicated in this dog?
iii. How would you treat this dog?

57 A 12-week-old crossbreed pup died 48 hours after the onset of severe haemorrhagic diarrhoea and vomiting. The pup was unvaccinated. On postmortem examination the small intestine was found to be congested (57) and the small intestinal contents were haemorrhagic.

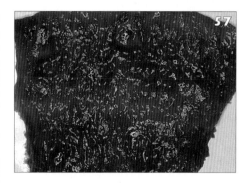

i. What viral agents would you consider as possible causes?
ii. What therapeutic options would you have considered if the pup had survived?
iii. What steps could you take to confirm your diagnosis?

56 i. The dog is jaundiced. Haemolysis is unlikely since the mucous membranes still have a pink tinge to them, and is ruled out by the normal PCV; the jaundice in this dog is therefore of hepatic or posthepatic origin. Low glucose and cholesterol concentrations indicate reduced hepatocellular synthesis, suggesting a hepatic cause. ALT and ALP increases are of the same magnitude, indicative of hepatocellular injury as well as cholestasis.

ii. Liver biopsy could be done to rule out other diseases and to define the prognosis; however, one should consider the possible benefits from this procedure in this case. Liver disease in this dog is likely to be acute, based on the short history, the absence of biochemical changes that might signify chronicity (such as hypoalbuminaemia) and the normal liver size. The history of anaesthesia coupled with antibiotic administration may suggest a hepatotoxic cause, especially since both agents are potentially hepatotoxic. In acute toxic liver disease, biopsy has limited usefulness but it is indicated if the dog does not readily improve on symptomatic therapy.

iii. Symptomatic treatment in this dog should consist of fluid therapy (to maintain liver perfusion), glucose supplementation in the drip (to combat hypoglycaemia), broad-spectrum antibiotics (to prevent secondary bacterial infection resulting from reduced hepatic reticuloendothelial system function) and vitamin B supplementation. Dietary protein need not be restricted if there is no evidence for hepatic encephalopathy, but it should be of high quality and highly digestible. Drugs such as ursodeoxycholic acid are not recommended in acute liver disease.

57 i. Canine parvovirus (CPV) and canine distemper virus infections are the most likely aetiological agents. Canine coronavirus infection rarely causes such clinical signs unless complicating factors such as concomitant infections with pathogenic bacteria or protozoal organisms are present. Canine rotavirus only causes mild GI signs in neonatal dogs.

ii. • Intravenous fluid therapy. If hypokalaemia or hypoglycaemia are present, the fluids may need to be supplemented with potassium or glucose.

• Prophylactic parenteral (not oral) broad-spectrum antibacterial drugs (e.g. clavulanate-potentiated amoxycillin) because of evidence of intestinal mucosal ulceration. Where there is evidence of septicaemia, gentamicin or cephalosporins are also indicated. In the absence of haemorrhage, antibacterials are not indicated.

• When there is evidence of GI ulceration, food should be withheld until the melena resolves (usually 24–48 hours). In the absence of GI bleeding it is not necessary to withhold food as long as a highly digestible diet is fed and feeding does not worsen the vomiting or fluid and electrolyte losses.

• In intractable cases where fluid losses cannot be managed with intravenous fluid therapy, opiates may be helpful in increasing gut transit time so as to reduce faecal fluid losses.

• Metoclopramide to control vomiting.

iii. Paired serology taken two weeks apart may be useful, depending upon when the samples were taken and which agent is present. Antibody levels rise quickly following CPV infection and moderate to high titres may already be present by the time clinical signs are seen. Histopathological examination of intestine, bone marrow, lymph node, brain and lung offers the best chance of making a diagnosis. Demonstration of viral antigen or virus isolation are useful during the acute phases of infection.

	Pre-anaesthetic	Day 7	Day 9	Day 23
Urea (mmol/l)	4.3	27.8	9.6	49
Creatinine (µmol/l)	8.0	309	168	619
Sodium (mmol/l)	148	147	149	144
Potassium (mmol/l)	4.5	4.2	4.3	5.2
Total CO_2 (mmol/l)	18	11	17	7
Calcium (mmol/l)	2.6	2.5	2.6	2.7
Phosphorus (mmol/l)	1.2	3.0	1.5	3.1
Amylase (u/l)	525	1,100	375	1,350
Urine SG	1.025	1.009	1.009	1.010
Urine protein	1+	2+	2+	3+
Urine casts	Negative	Negative	Negative	Negative
Urine sediment	Negative	Inactive	Inactive	Inactive

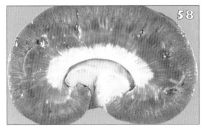

58 A 14-year-old, neutered female Samoyed is anaesthetized for routine dentistry and excision of several cutaneous and subcutaneous masses. She has degenerative joint disease (DJD) in multiple joints and hip dysplasia, and is receiving aspirin (14 mg/kg q12h). Pre-anaesthetic blood work-up is shown. Anaesthesia is induced with ketamine and midazolam, and maintained with isoflurane. Lactated Ringer's solution is administered (2.2 ml/kg/hr) during the procedure. She recovers uneventfully. The masses are sebaceous adenomas and lipomas. Seven days later the dog is depressed, polyuric/polydipsic and 5% dehydrated. The incisions are healing normally. Biochemistry results are shown. After 48 hours of fluid therapy laboratory evaluation is repeated (day 9 results). Fluid therapy is discontinued over the next 48 hours. The dog is eating and drinking and is released from the hospital. Two weeks later the dog is readmitted because she has been vomiting for two days. Laboratory evaluation is repeated (day 23 results). The owners elect for euthanasia. Necropsy revealed glomerular amyloidosis, acute tubular necrosis (renal papillary necrosis) (58), DJD of multiple joints and fibrosis at the surgical incision.

i. What is your interpretation of the data up to and including day 7?
ii. What is oliguria? If the dog is oliguric after rehydration, what can be done to attempt conversion to non-oliguria?
iii. What does the finding of acute tubular necrosis (ATN) imply?
iv. What pathophysiological mechanisms may have resulted in ATN?
v. What might have been done differently?

59 You have diagnosed insulinoma in a ten-year-old dog. How would you treat this case?

58 i. Azotaemia with isosthenuria indicates primary renal failure. Because the blood work-up was normal one week previously, the renal failure is probably acute in nature.

ii. Oliguria is defined as urine production <0.5 ml/kg/hr. If oliguria is present after rehydration, there are several strategies to attempt to convert oliguria to non-oliguria including: frusemide (2.2–17 mg/kg i/v); dopamine administered with frusemide (1–3 mg/kg/minute i/v); mannitol (0.5–1 g/kg of a 10–20% solution as a slow bolus i/v); dextrose in water (10–20% dextrose at 25–50 ml/kg over 1–2 hours). These protocols may be alternated with lactated Ringer's solution.

iii. Acute renal failure, probably as a result of acute tubular necrosis.

iv. Acute tubular necrosis (renal papillary necrosis) may result from a toxic or ischaemic event to the renal tubules. Although NSAIDs are not nephrotoxic when used at appropriate dosages, their use may contribute to the development of acute renal failure when other risk factors are present. NSAIDs may potentiate the risk for acute tubular necrosis during periods of hypotension or hypovolaemia. Other risk factors include age, fever, volume depletion, pre-existing renal disease, liver disease, hypokalaemia, hypomagnesaemia, nephrotoxins, other causes of reduced renal perfusion and sepsis. These risk factors are additive in effect.

v. In retrospect the dog was proteinuric (1+ protein with a SG of 1.025). Urine had been saved from the pre-anaesthetic examination and the urine protein:creatinine ratio was 5:1. Pending additional work-up, dentistry and mass excisional surgery may have been delayed. More aggressive fluid therapy during anaesthesia and post-operatively may have been undertaken. Lastly, alternative analgesics may have been administered and NSAIDs could have been discontinued for a couple of weeks prior to the anaesthetic episode.

59 Surgical removal is the treatment of choice for single masses. Where metastasis has occurred, debulking is recommended as this makes medical management easier. To reduce the frequency and severity of clinical signs and to avoid acute hypoglycaemic crises, frequent feeding of a diet high in protein, fat and complex carbohydrates is recommended. Simple sugars, honey, syrup and chocolate should be avoided. Exercise should be limited to short walks. Prednisolone can be used once dietary therapy fails, as it antagonizes the effects of insulin, thereby indirectly increasing blood glucose, and promotes hepatic glycogenolysis, thereby directly increasing blood glucose. Marked weight gain is common in treated animals. Diazoxide inhibits insulin secretion, stimulates hepatic gluconeogenesis and glycogenolysis, and inhibits tissue use of glucose. The net result is to increase blood glucose concentrations. Diazoxide does not inhibit insulin synthesis and it is not cytotoxic.

60 A one-year-old, female German Shorthaired Pointer has had clinical signs of oestrus and male attractiveness for 45 days. The bitch is clinically well. Examination of a vaginal smear shows the presence of 75% anuclear cells and an absence of neutrophils. An ultrasound examination of the ovaries has been performed and an image obtained of the left ovary (60).

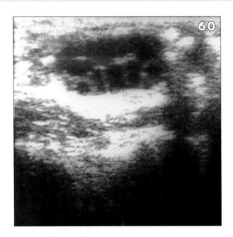

i. What is your diagnosis?
ii. How common is this condition, and what are the differential diagnoses?
iii. How might this condition be treated?
iv. What is the likely chance of recurrence, and the significance for fertility?

61 A four-year-old Siamese cat is presented with an 18-month history of intermittent vomiting, which usually occurs several hours after feeding. The vomitus generally contains partially digested food.
i. What are your differential diagnoses?

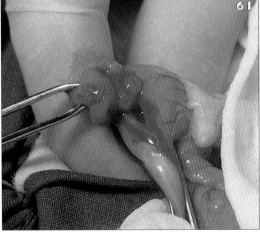

Per-oral gastroscopy and duodenoscopy reveal a mass protruding into the proximal small intestine. Exploratory laparotomy and enterotomy reveal a pedunculated mass (61).
ii. What is the probable diagnosis in this cat, and what is the prognosis?

60 i. The ultrasound image shows an enlarged ovary with multiple anechoic structures of varying shape and size present throughout the stroma. This appearance is consistent with follicular cysts. Follicular cysts produce oestrogen and are usually associated with clinical signs of persistent oestrus. In some bitches the persistent elevation of oestrogen (hyperoestrogenism) can cause bone marrow suppression resulting in anaemia and thrombocytopenia. This ovary can be distinguished from a normal oestrus ovary because the latter generally has a smaller number of follicles of similar size. Follicles normally increase in size and ovulate when they reach approximately 11 mm in diameter.

ii. True follicular cysts are rare in the bitch. Cysts associated with the ovary are common, but these are usually present within the ovarian bursa and are not endocrinologically active and therefore produce no clinical signs. Differential diagnoses of oestrogen-producing follicular cysts are those bitches with a long proestrus and/or oestrus and bitches with split oestrus syndrome. The former may not ovulate until as late as 30 days after the onset of proestrus and the latter generally have an absence of oestrous signs before a return at some future time; in both cases the ovaries are ultrasonographically normal. Some ovarian tumours may produce oestrogen and produce clinical signs of persistent oestrus. These bitches are usually systemically unwell and have ascites.

iii. It may be possible to induce either ovulation or luteinization of follicular cysts by the administration of human chorionic gonadotrophin. If successful, the bitch enters metoestrus and has a normal interoestrous interval of approximately seven months. If this treatment is not successful, exogenous progestogens may be used to suppress the follicles and cause a resolution of the clinical signs. In some cases, oestrus and ovulation follow shortly after progestogen withdrawal, whilst in others the interoestrous interval is delayed for up to four months.

iv. After successful therapy or, occasionally, spontaneous regression, bitches frequently return to normal cyclicity with no reduction in fertility.

61 i. Vomiting of partially digested food several hours after feeding suggests a gastric outflow obstruction. Pyloric dysfunction would probably be the most likely diagnosis in this individual as it is recognized as a particular problem in Siamese cats. In this breed it is sometimes seen in association with megaoesophagus, and appears to be a functional abnormality rather than true pyloric stenosis. Other differential diagnoses would include true pyloric stenosis, primary or secondary gastric motility disorders, inflammatory bowel disease, chronic gastritis (e.g. secondary to *Ollulanus tricuspis* infection), gastric or duodenal neoplasia, and gastric or duodenal polyps.

ii. The pedunculated nature of this mass is typical of a benign duodenal polyp, although histological examination would be required to rule out neoplasia. Benign adenomatous duodenal polyps are an uncommon problem but several cases have been reported in cats. A longitudinal enterotomy incision through the antemesenteric border of the duodenum to expose the mass allows excision of the polyp at its base in the duodenal mucosa. Excision is curative, with no recurrences reported. Although typically located in the proximal duodenum, some of the adenomatous masses appear to represent ectopic gastric tissue, whereas others are composed of duodenal tissue. In addition to duodenal polyps, ileal polyps have also been reported in Siamese cats.

62 A 16-week-old, unvaccinated male Rottweiler puppy is
presented with a two-day history of anorexia, lethargy and
vomiting, and a one-day history of collapse and haemorrhagic diarrhoea (62a). On physical
examination the rectal temperature is 37.5°C (98.6°F) and
the heart rate is 165 bpm; the
puppy is assessed as 10% dehydrated, based on skin turgor. Despite intensive fluid

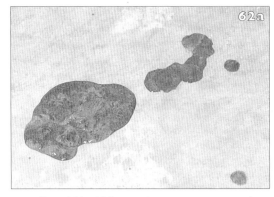

therapy and supportive care the puppy dies within 12 hours. At postmortem examination the intestines are haemorrhagic with diffuse erosions. You strongly suspect canine
parvovirus (CPV) infection.
i. List at least four other major differential diagnoses.
ii. Describe how you would confirm the diagnosis of CPV infection.

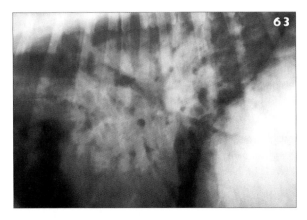

63 A six-month-old, unvaccinated crossbreed dog is presented with acute onset
haemorrhagic diarrhoea, vomiting, dyspnoea and a mucopurulent nasal discharge.
Auscultation of the chest reveals harsh crackles and an overall increase in lung
sounds. Auscultation of the heart is unremarkable. Abdominal pain is present.
Mucous membranes are pale and the dog is depressed. A thoracic radiograph is taken
(63).
i. How would you interpret this radiograph?
ii. What viral disorder would you consider most likely in this dog?
iii. How might you confirm your diagnosis?

62 i. Viral enteritides (CPV*, distemper, infectious canine hepatitis); haemorrhagic gastroenteritis (HGE)*; garbage enteritis*; hypoadrenocorticism*; acute bacterial enteritis (salmonellosis*, shigellosis, campylobacteriosis); intestinal obstruction (intussusception*, foreign body, strangulated hernia); poisoning (anticoagulants); para-

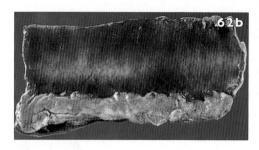

sitism (*Ancylostoma*). (*Diagnoses of major importance.)

ii. The age and vaccinal status of this dog would raise suspicions of an infectious disease, and history of contact with other affected dogs would be an important clue. The clinical signs and characteristic time course of 'dull the first day, vomiting on the second, diarrhoea on the third and dead or better on the fourth' are suggestive of CPV infection. Pyrexia is expected after initial CPV infection but this puppy was *in extremis* and hypothermic when presented, probably secondary to endotoxic shock. Hypovolaemic shock and hypothermia may also be seen with hypoadrenocorticism or with HGE. Other signs such as bradycardia, ill thrift and weight loss might be expected with hypoadrenocorticism. With HGE a markedly raised haematocrit (>0.65 l/l) but normal skin turgor in the face of massive loss of extracellular fluid into the intestine is characteristic. With CPV infection the haematocrit may be slightly elevated and a leucopenia may be present. If necessary, perform radiography and ultrasound examination. Bacteriology is indicated to rule out salmonellosis. Antemortem diagnosis of CPV infection can be confirmed by serology or identification of viral antigen in faeces by ELISA or haemagglutinin assay. Paired serology is impossible in this case, but peak antibody titre is reached rapidly and, although death occurred early, some serological response is likely to be evident. Virus isolation may be attempted on intestinal contents. The postmortem appearance (**62b**) (enlarged mesenteric lymph nodes, a granular serosal surface and a denuded mucosal surface with floccules of mucosal debris and often little blood) is not immediately suggestive of intestinal infection, but histology (epithelial sloughing, villous necrosis and crypt dilation) is sufficient to confirm the diagnosis.

63 i. The radiograph shows a mixed bronchial and alveolar pattern in all lung lobes. Air bronchograms and alveolar consolidation are evident. Extrapulmonary tissues are unremarkable. The radiographic diagnosis is of a bronchopneumonia.
ii. Canine distemper virus (CDV) infection.
iii. CDV infection is difficult to confirm. The organism is difficult to isolate. Cytoplasmic inclusion bodies in epithelial cells from the cornea or bladder wall would be suggestive of CDV. A rising antibody titre on paired serum samples taken three weeks apart would also indicate an active CDV infection.

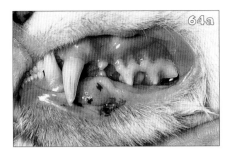
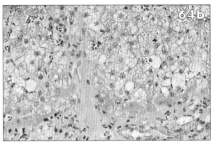

64 A four-year-old, neutered male, indoor domestic shorthair cat became inappetent soon after the owners moved in to a new home and obtained a puppy. The cat initially weighed 7.6 kg but within two weeks had lost 1.3 kg. On physical examination he was quiet, in fair body condition and markedly jaundiced (64a). The rounded, caudal edge of the liver could be palpated beyond the costochondral junction. Pertinent laboratory findings included: PCV 0.42 l/l, ALP 522 u/l, ALT 168 u/l, GGT 2 u/l, total bilirubin 145 µmol/l and fasting bile acids 123 µmol/l. A liver biopsy was obtained (64b).

i. What is your diagnosis?

ii. What are some of the predisposing factors of this condition for which this cat should be evaluated?

iii. What are the important factors in the treatment of this condition?

65 A ten-year-old, neutered male cat presented with acute onset collapse, very pale mucous membranes and abdominal distension. Physical examination revealed an enlarged liver. Thoracic auscultation and peripheral lymph nodes were unremarkable. On abdominal paracentesis, blood was obtained which failed to clot on standing. Abdominal radiography demonstrated a large liver. Ultrasonography revealed numerous small hypoechoic

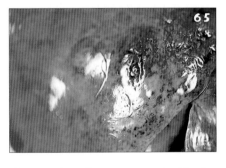

areas within the liver parenchyma. Haematology confirmed severe anaemia. Platelet numbers were adequate and a coagulation screen was normal. Clinical biochemistry showed mild increases in ALT and ALP. The liver contained multiple haemorrhagic areas below the capsule (65). Some had ruptured causing the haemoabdomen. At postmortem examination the lesions noted in the liver were not found elsewhere in the cat.

i. What are your main differential diagnoses for haemoabdomen prior to performing any diagnostic work-up?

ii. What is your presumptive diagnosis pending histopathology?

64 i. The appearance of vacuolated hepatocytes in conjunction with the history of anorexia and weight loss support a diagnosis of hepatic lipidosis. The laboratory findings of a moderately elevated serum ALP activity in conjunction with a normal serum GGT activity can also be a clue, for this serum liver enzyme pattern is a characteristic finding in affected cats. An Oil-Red-O stain for lipids would confirm that the non-stained material within the hepatocytes is indeed lipid.

ii. In approximately 50% of cases, hepatic lipidosis is secondary to another underlying disease process. The most common concurrent and/or causative diseases include diabetes mellitus, cholangiohepatitis, pancreatitis, renal disease, hyperthyroidism, neoplasia, cardiomyopathy and other systemic illnesses that result in anorexia for five days or longer. Idiopathic hepatic lipidosis (IHL) is a diagnosis of exclusion when no other underlying disease can be identified. Therefore, a thorough laboratory analysis including viral titres and endocrine function tests, as well as diagnostic imaging studies, are needed to rule out a primary disease process. Common denominating factors in animals that develop IHL seem to be a sedentary lifestyle, obesity and subsequent anorexia in association with an environmental stress such as changing home, or the introduction of a new, unfamiliar animal as in this cat's history.

iii. Adequate protein-calorie nutrition is the cornerstone of therapy for the treatment of hepatic lipidosis. Although the underlying pathogenesis of hepatic lipidosis remains unknown, it appears that in times of excess ketogenesis, such as starvation, the feline liver lacks the ability to mobilize the excessively accumulating lipids, the hepatocytes become inundated with fat vacuoles, and a vicious cycle of anorexia and worsening liver function ensues. Since it is difficult to get these animals to eat an adequate amount of calories, and force feeding is rarely successful, the placement of a gastric feeding tube and the feeding of a moderate- to high-protein diet has improved the survival rate of cats affected with IHL significantly. The addition of essential amino acids such as carnitine, arginine and taurine have been advocated to assist in the mobilization of lipids from hepatocytes and the recovery of normal liver function.

65 i. Coagulopathies; neoplasia – haemangiosarcoma, vascular tumour; thrombosis; torsion – spleen, stomach; trauma; tumour eroding a vessel; vascular anomaly. In the cat all of these, with the exception of trauma, are rare.

ii. The appearance of the liver was consistent with peliosis hepatis. The diagnosis was confirmed on histopathology. This term is used to designate focal, blood-filled spaces in the liver. It resembles telangiectasis. The cause of the lesions is unknown. They may be present as asymptomatic lesions, but if they are extensive and rupture, severe blood loss results.

66 An eight-month-old, female Cocker Spaniel is presented because of a progressive enlargement of the clitoris which now protrudes from the vulval orifice (66). Examination shows that the vulva is small and somewhat cranially positioned. Palpation of the clitoris demonstrates that it has a central bone.
i. What is the likely diagnosis?
ii. What is the aetiology of this condition?
iii. What are the treatment options?

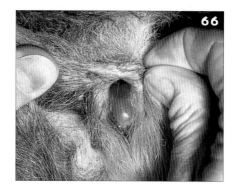

67 A six-year-old, male Doberman Pinscher is evaluated for lethargy and decreased appetite of two weeks' duration. An enlarged liver is palpated and an ultrasonogram is subsequently obtained (67).
i. What are the differential diagnoses for hepatomegaly?
ii. What abnormality do you see on this hepatic ultrasonogram?
iii. How would you proceed from here?

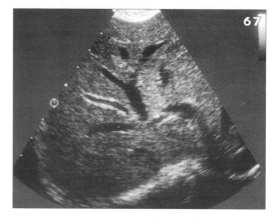

68 A young dog presented with a long-term history of intermittent vomiting, regurgitation and hypersalivation. The vomiting occurred at variable times after eating. The dog was well grown, bright and keen to eat. Diarrhoea was not a feature. Occasional coughing was reported. A chest radiograph was taken after administration of barium (68).
i. What is your diagnosis?
ii. What further diagnostic tests would you recommend?
iii. What treatment would you recommend for your likely diagnosis?

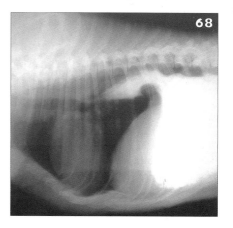

66 i. This bitch is an intersex. The time of onset of the clinical signs corresponds with the onset of puberty and it is likely that there is androgen production by gonadal testicular tissue. Androgens (predominantly testosterone) cause clitoral enlargement and development of an os clitoris. Frequently there is excessive licking of the vulva due to low-grade vestibulitis.

ii. Intersex animals may be classified according to the following three abnormalities:
• Abnormalities of chromosomal sex – sex chromosome aneuploids, chimeras or mosaics. These phenotypic females with underdeveloped genitalia develop changes in the clitoris at puberty. The recognition of abnormalities of chromosomal sex requires the construction of a karyotype.
• Abnormalities of gonadal sex – chromosomal and gonadal sex do not agree. These are the so-called sex-reversed animals where there is translocation of the Tdy antigen onto the X chromosome or an autosome. Of the three categories of this condition, only one presents with an externally female phenotypic reproductive tract. They are true hermaphrodites with ovotestes, oviducts and external female genitalia.
• Abnormalities of phenotypic sex – females which have ovaries and XX chromosomes (female pseudohermaphrodites). These are masculinized due to exposure to exogenous or endogenous androgens *in utero*.

iii. The majority of intersex animals are infertile and surgical neutering is the preferred method of treatment. Following removal of the gonads, the os clitoris may become smaller as the animal grows and the clinical signs resolve. Clitoridectomy is mostly unnecessary but after puberty the clitoris may be large and require surgical removal.

67 i. Hepatomegaly may be due to infiltrative liver disease (neoplasia, amyloidosis), excessive storage (lipidosis, glycogen), severe congestion, diffuse inflammation (in the dog only with acute inflammation; in the cat with both acute and chronic inflammation), nodular hyperplasia or work hypertrophy.

ii. The liver looks congested with markedly distended portal vein branches, suggesting congestive heart failure or posthepatic venous obstruction.

iii. Evaluate the cardiovascular system. Doberman Pinschers are prone to cardiomyopathy; myocardial fractional shortening may be evaluated via echocardiography. Angiographic contrast studies may be needed to assess posthepatic venous obstruction.

68 i. The radiograph shows reflux of barium into the oesophagus, an appearance typical of a disorder of the oesophageal hiatus, i.e. a hiatal hernia.

ii. Fluoroscopy may demonstrate the presence of a sliding hiatal hernia. Direct abdominal pressure or manually obstructing the upper airway improves the likelihood of demonstrating an intermittent problem. Endoscopy may reveal oesophagitis supporting a diagnosis of gastro-oesophageal reflux. View the lower oesophageal sphincter from the gastric side; gastric insufflation may cause cranial displacement of the cardia.

iii. Cimetidine or ranitidine to block acid production. Sucralfate is useful as a mucosal protectant. Metoclopramide or cisapride increases the tone of the gastro-oesophageal junction and promotes gastric emptying. If there is upper airway disease or obesity, this should be corrected. Severe cases require surgery.

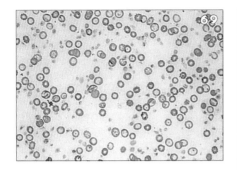

RBCs ($\times 10^{12}$/l)	2.61
Hb (g/l)	• 35
PCV (l/l)	0.18
MCV (fl)	68
MCHC (g/l)	200
nRBCs	7%
Platelets ($\times 10^9$/l)	1,320
WBCs ($\times 10^9$/l)	26.8
Neutrophils (seg) ($\times 10^9$/l)	16.3
Neutrophils (bands) ($\times 10^9$/l)	4.56
Lymphocytes ($\times 10^9$/l)	1.61
Monocytes ($\times 10^9$/l)	2.14
Eosinophils ($\times 10^9$/l)	0.27

69 A middle-aged Collie-cross presents with pallor and reduced exercise tolerance. The haematological findings and a photomicrograph (**69**) of the blood film are shown.

i. What is your comment on the film? Note the RBC and platelet morphology.
ii. How would you interpret the haematological findings?
iii. What further questions might you ask the owner?
iv. How would you confirm your suspicions?

70 An 11-month-old, unvaccinated Border Collie presented with acute onset epileptiform fits of one-half to two minutes' duration (**70**). Between fits the dog was quadriparetic but otherwise bright. Cranial nerve examination showed sluggish pupillary light reflexes; otherwise no abnormalities were noted. His rectal temperature was 39.5°C (103.1°F). He had been treated for acute upper respiratory tract infection, vomiting and haemorrhagic diarrhoea two months previously, which had resolved after two weeks. There were no previous reports of neurological signs. The dog was not a scavenger and had not knowingly been exposed to toxic materials.

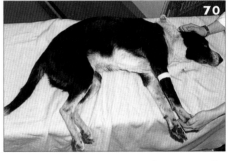

i. What diagnoses would you consider?
ii. What diagnostic plan would you recommend, and what abnormalities might you expect to find for the different diagnoses you have considered?

69 i. The film confirms the platelet count (normally in the dog 8–29 platelets per ×100 oil immersion field). Platelet anisocytosis, polychromasia ++, RBC anisocytosis - and hypochromia ++ are noted.

ii. This is a marked hypochromic and normocytic anaemia. The polychromasia suggests strong regeneration and despite this the MCV is not increased. There is a thrombocytosis, a neutrophilia with a left shift and a monocytosis. The WBC counts would be consistent with inflammation or infection, but are more likely to reflect non-specific bone marrow stimulation associated with regenerative activity. Both thrombocytosis and hypochromic anaemia are typically present in iron deficiency. The commonest cause of iron deficiency in adult dogs is chronic GI haemorrhage from tumours, inflammatory bowel disease or hookworm parasitism. This profile probably reflects a regenerative response to blood loss in the face of chronic iron deficiency.

iii. Establish the worming history and whether dark faeces or melena had been seen.

iv. Confirmation of iron deficiency requires an iron profile. Measurement of serum ferritin might also be useful.

70 i. • Canine distemper virus (CDV) infection is likely given the previous history. CDV may also cause dermatological changes (hyperkeratosis). Different CDV strains show differing pathogenicities and organ tropisms, with some only causing clinical disease in one or two organ systems. The development of neurological signs associated with CDV is often delayed in onset.

• Inherited or acquired epilepsy.

• A form of inflammatory meningoencephalitis.

• Toxicity, e.g. lead, organophosphates. Lead poisoning may cause GI signs, although the time interval between the development of GI signs and CNS signs in this case would be unusual.

ii. • Haematology may reflect the presence of an inflammatory disorder. Basophilic stippling of RBCs would be indicative of lead poisoning. Acute CDV infection may cause a leucopenia, although it would be highly unlikely that this would still be in evidence two months after the initial infection. Haematology was unremarkable in this case.

• Clinical biochemistry may be helpful if a toxicity is suspected. Assessment of renal and hepatic parameters is indicated as well as blood lead levels. In this dog the biochemistry was unremarkable.

• CSF analysis. The CSF contained 35 g/l protein, a CDV antibody titre of 1:1600 (titre in serum was 1:400) and a WBC count of 2.5×10^9/l, comprising 50% non-degenerate neutrophils, 40% lymphocytes and 10% macrophages. The high CDV antibody titre in CSF compared to plasma would suggest active CDV infection in the CNS. The increased protein content and WBC count are consistent with an inflammatory disorder.

71 A four-year-old, male crossbreed dog presented for inappetence, weight loss and occasional vomiting of several weeks' duration. Clinical pathology revealed hyperglobulinaemia (52 g/l), hypoalbuminaemia (19 g/l) and elevated liver enzymes (ALT 800 u/l, ALP 950 u/l). Urinalysis showed a SG of 1.024, trace protein and 2+ bilirubin. Fasting serum bile acids were 140 µmol/l. Abdominal radiography revealed reduced liver size. A liver biopsy showed severe chronic hepatitis with marked periportal accumulation of mononuclear inflammatory cells which were invading the hepatic lobule and infiltrating the hepatic parenchyma.

How might you treat this case?

72 A two-year-old, neutered female Cocker Spaniel has been polyuric, polydipsic, vomiting and inappetent for several weeks. Routine laboratory investigations revealed the abnormalities shown. A left lateral radiograph of the abdomen is obtained (72).

PCV (l/l)	0.24
Reticulocytes (%)	0.2
Urea (mmol/l)	54.2
Creatinine (µmol/l)	389
Phosphorus (mmol/l)	9.44
Calcium (mmol/l)	2.35

i. Describe your radiographic findings.
ii. What is your diagnosis?
iii. What can be done medically to help relieve the signs of gastritis?

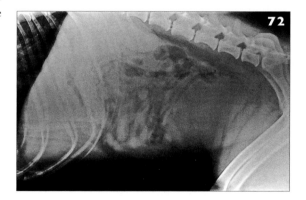

71 Slowing the progression of disease, managing the metabolic consequences and providing an optimum environment for hepatic regeneration. Initial treatment:
• Corticosteroids (2 mg/kg/day, gradually tapering) modulate the inflammatory and fibrotic response in chronic hepatitis. They have the disadvantage of being catabolic, contraindicating their use in animals with hepatic encephalopathy, while high doses may cause a reversible hepatopathy. They are particularly indicated in this patient because of the severity of inflammation. Tapering doses and long-term alternate day treatment are preferred. Follow-up biopsies may be required to assess the efficacy of treatment, since biochemical re-evaluation is hampered by steroid-induced enzyme induction (especially ALP). Treatment response to glucocorticoids may be suspected based on improvement of clinical signs, serum ALT activity and liver function tests. For patients that fail to respond to corticosteroid therapy alone, prednisolone may be combined at a reduced dose with azathioprine (1–2 mg/kg daily or every other day).
• Ursodeoxycholic acid (10–15 mg/kg q24h). A hydrophilic bile acid which protects hepatocytes by displacing toxic hydrophobic bile acids, but also has choleretic and immunomodulatory properties. It should be used in conjunction with other measures aimed at controlling the pathogenesis of the disease.
• A high-quality protein diet with micronutrient supplementation. Frequent feeding of a diet providing adequate calories (carbohydrates and lipids), protein and micronutrients (B vitamins, zinc) is important to support hepatocyte regeneration. Adequate calories (1.25–1.5 × MER) should be fed, since patients are often catabolic and in negative nitrogen balance. Frequent feeding of small meals reduces fasting hypoglycaemia and increases protein tolerance. Protein should be of high quality and digestibility in order to minimize nitrogenous waste production. Excessive restriction of dietary protein may be harmful by worsening hypoalbuminaemia. Fat is a good source of energy and restriction of dietary fat is only indicated in dogs with severe cholestasis and steatorrhoea. Maintenance requirements for water soluble B-complex vitamins should be doubled since these frequently become deficient in liver disease, but supplementation with other vitamins should be done with caution. Zinc supplementation (zinc sulphate 2 mg/kg/day or zinc gluconate 3 mg/kg/day) is recommended.

72 i. The gastric mucosa is more diffusely radiopaque with prominent, well-defined rugal folds representing probable soft tissue mineralization.
ii. The long-standing clinical signs, azotaemia and non-regenerative anaemia indicate that this dog is in chronic renal failure. Many animals with renal failure experience vomiting and inappetence due to the retention of gastrin, resultant gastric hyperacidity and the influence of uraemic toxins. In this dog the mineralization seen in the gastric wall is likely a result of persistent, severe elevations in serum phosphorus concentrations which complex with calcium and may precipitate in soft tissues, such as the stomach and kidneys, and exacerbate the clinical signs of uraemia. The diagnosis is chronic renal failure with a calcified, uraemic gastropathy.
iii. The soft tissue mineralization is irreversible, but the variables that can be manipulated include decreasing serum phosphate concentrations with a diet low in phosphorus, administering phosphate binders with meals, and controlling gastric acidity with histamine blockers and other gastric protectant medications.

	Middle-aged Cocker Spaniel	Aged Labrador	Reference range
Serum iron (SI) (ml/dl)	50	50	84–233
Unbound iron binding capacity (UIBC) (µl/dl)	350	150	142–393
Total iron binding capacity (TIBC) (µl/dl)	400	200	284–572
Saturation (%)	12.5	25	20–59

73 Interpret the iron profiles above obtained from two dogs with chronic anaemia. One has iron deficiency anaemia and the other anaemia of chronic disease associated with an inflammatory disorder. Which is which?

74 This ultrasonogram (74) is of a 12-year-old, male German Shepherd Dog presented with sudden onset lethargy and collapse. He is recumbent and has pale mucous membranes and a rapid thready pulse (160 bpm). The abdomen feels slightly fluctuant. Abdominal radiographs show some peritoneal fluid and paracentesis yields a small amount of blood.

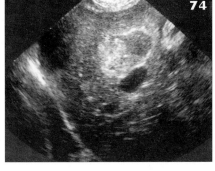

i. What are your differential diagnoses?
ii. What could be the reason for performing abdominal ultrasonography?
iii. What abnormality do you see on this hepatic ultrasonogram?

75 You perform a retrograde urethrogram (75) as part of the work-up of a male dog with haematuria.
i. Describe how you would perform such a procedure?
ii. What is your interpretation of this radiograph?
iii. What are the main features that you would be looking for when assessing retrograde urethrograms?

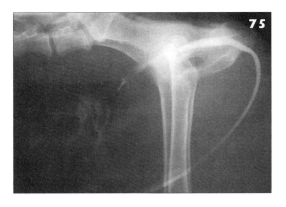

73 The values of significance are SI, TIBC and percentage saturation. UIBC is a direct measurement used to calculate TIBC (TIBC = SI + UIBC). Iron deficiency is characterized by low serum iron, low saturation and normal TIBC. Anaemia of chronic disease has normal to low serum iron, low TIBC and normal to low saturation. The low TIBC in inflammation is due to altered hepatic synthesis of plasma proteins which results in reduced transferrin and albumin synthesis, and increased synthesis of acute phase proteins such as haptoglobin, ceruloplasmin and fibrinogen. The middle-aged Cocker Spaniel is iron deficient and the aged Labrador has anaemia of chronic disease. Clearly, measuring serum iron alone would not discriminate between these causes of non-regenerative anaemia.

74 i. The dog has a haemoabdomen and appears to be in haemorrhagic shock. Causes of haemoabdomen include a ruptured neoplasm (especially haemangiosarcoma), traumatic rupture and coagulopathy. In the absence of trauma and with no evidence for a bleeding problem, splenic haemangiosarcoma is a major differential in this breed.
ii. Radiography does not necessarily demonstrate small intra-abdominal lesions, and this may be especially difficult if there is free abdominal fluid. Abdominal ultrasonography is a more sensitive technique to look for parenchymatous lesions.
iii. The ultrasonogram shows abdominal fluid (blood) surrounding the liver and a large hyperechoic and cavitating lesion within the liver, suggestive of neoplasia. No other abdominal abnormalities were found. The owners elected for euthanasia. At postmortem examination, metastatic hepatic haemangiosarcoma was found to be the cause of the abdominal haemorrhage.

75 i. Prior to the procedure the colon and rectum should be emptied of all faecal material, using an oral laxative administered for the previous two days or an enema administered the afternoon and morning prior to anaesthesia. Retrograde urethrography, plain radiography and negative contrast cystography should be carried out first. For retrograde urethrography a urinary catheter (the largest that will pass comfortably) is inserted to just beyond the os penis. The prepuce is lightly clamped around the catheter to reduce any back flow of contrast material onto the table, and contrast material is administered through the catheter to fill the urethra. For a 30 kg dog, approximately 25 ml of a water-soluble contrast agent is injected and the film exposed as the last 5 ml is administered. When positioning the dog, be sure that the whole of the urethra is included; lateral recumbency is required. Before injection the bladder should contain some air.
ii. This radiograph is unremarkable.
iii. The main features which would be considered abnormal are narrowing/obstruction to contrast flow along the urethra, the presence of filling defects in the contrast column, roughening of the urethral mucosa, and leakage of contrast material into the prostate. It is normal for the urethra to be slightly narrowed as it passes around the ischial arch and for the intrapelvic urethra to be wider.

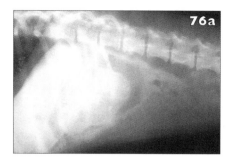

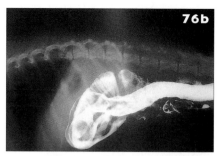

76 A two-year-old Jack Russell Terrier presented with a history of chronic intermittent vomiting and diarrhoea of 18 months' duration. Vomiting occurred from one to several hours after eating and was predominantly food. The diarrhoea was of variable consistency (water to pasty). Neither blood nor mucus was present in the diarrhoea. The bitch had never gained weight and was thin. Her appetite was normal and she was bright, alert and responsive. A slight increase in the frequency of defecation was reported when diarrhoea was evident. A non-painful linear soft tissue mass (3 cm × 4 cm) was palpable in the cranial abdomen. All other body systems appeared normal.

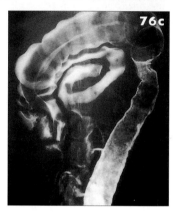

i. What are your main differential diagnoses?
   Abdominal radiographs were taken (76a–76c).
ii. What is your interpretation of these radiographs?
iii. What is the cause of the condition you have identified?

77 A three-year-old, female Bedlington Terrier presented for intermittent vomiting of two months' duration. The dog would vomit two to three times a week and the vomiting did not follow any pattern. Recently the dog had started to lose some weight. Physical examination revealed an alert dog in fair body condition (77a). A serum biochemical profile revealed only

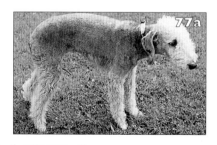

moderately elevated liver enzymes (ALT 315 u/l, ALP 287 u/l).
i. What are your differential diagnoses?
ii. What is the significance of your laboratory findings?
iii. How would you proceed from here?

76 i. The nature of the diarrhoea (absence of blood and mucus) and absence of weight gain would suggest small intestinal disease. Vomiting suggests gastric or intestinal disease. The major differential diagnoses considered were IBD, SIBO, chronic partial intestinal obstruction, chronic intussusception and dietary intolerance. The non-painful, sausage-shaped soft tissue mass was most consistent with intussusception.

ii. Plain radiography shows a well-defined soft tissue mass in the cranial abdomen. The barium study shows a dilated large intestine in the cranial abdomen immediately caudal to the stomach. The caecum contains a soft tissue mass with barium evident between this mass and the caecal mucosa and also present as a thin streak passing down the centre of the mass; this barium is in the lumen of the intussuscepted ileum. The appearance of the intestine is similar to that of a clock spring, in this case an ileocolic intussusception.

iii. Intussusceptions are thought to result from underlying disease which damages the wall of the intestine and locally inhibits normal propulsive and segmental motility. As a peristaltic wave passes along the gut, the intestine proximal to the damaged portion contracts over it and envelops it. They may develop as a sequela to parasitism, viral infection, linear foreign bodies, intestinal tumours or adhesions.

77 i. Causes of chronic vomiting outside the GI tract should be considered first (pyometra, liver disease, renal failure, hypoadrenocorticism, ketoacidotic diabetes mellitus, pancreatitis, peritonitis, drugs and toxins, CNS disease). These can be ruled out by history taking, physical examination and laboratory tests. Thereafter, possible gastric and/or intestinal causes of vomiting should be considered.

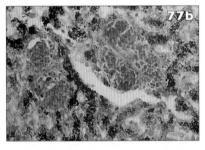

ii. Elevated liver enzymes in this dog suggest liver disease, but it is important to remember that liver enzyme elevations may be transient and may occur secondary to diseases outside the liver. Due to its central place in the metabolism the liver frequently becomes involved in disease elsewhere (the 'innocent bystander' phenomenon). However, the degree of ALT elevation is more than would be expected, and in a Bedlington Terrier it should alert the clinician to the possibility of copper hepatotoxicosis. This disease is common in the breed, and in early stages may only manifest itself by elevations in serum ALT.

iii. Measure serum bile acid concentrations and if these are increased, liver imaging and biopsy should be considered. If serum bile acids are normal, liver enzymes should be repeated after three and six weeks. If enzymes remain elevated, biopsy is indicated. Plain histology showed mild focal hepatitis, whereas the rhodanine stain for copper was strongly positive. The photomicrograph (**77b**) (rhodanine stain, ×25 original magnification) shows many dark-staining granules representing copper-loaded lysosomes. Copper overload can be confirmed via quantitative analysis. Treatment with de-coppering agents (such as D-penicillamine at 15 mg/kg q12h) is indicated in this dog. Treatment usually has to be given for months to years. Repeat liver biopsies should be performed to assess the efficacy of de-coppering.

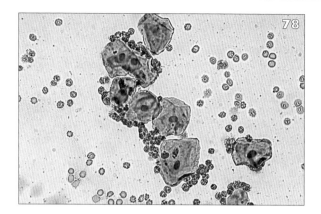

78 A three-year-old, female Collie-cross had a routine ovariohysterectomy at 18 months of age. Since that time she has had clinical signs of oestrus approximately every seven months and has been attractive to male dogs. Presently she has a red-tinged vulval discharge. A vaginal smear has been obtained and stained with a modified Wright-Giemsa stain (78).

i. What are the features of the vaginal smear, and what is the likely diagnosis?
ii. What techniques could be used to confirm this diagnosis?
iii. What are the differential diagnoses for this condition?
iv. How should the condition be treated?

79 An aged cat presented with an acute onset muscle weakness and ventroflexion of the neck. The cat was reported to have been polyuric and polydipsic for several weeks. There was no indication of depression or inappetence. Serum biochemistry findings are shown. Urine SG was 1.014.

Potassium (mmol/l)	2.8
Sodium (mmol/l)	145
Chloride (mmol/l)	120
Urea (mmol/l)	17.9
Creatinine (µmol/l)	240
ALT (u/l)	70
ALP (u/l)	80
Glucose (mmol/l)	10.6

i. How would you interpret these findings?
ii. What clinical/metabolic features may result from the hypokalaemia?
iii. How would you treat the electrolyte abnormality?

78 i. Both large and small intermediate epithelial cells and some erythrocytes are present within the smear. These changes are associated with an elevation in plasma oestrogen concentration, and the likely diagnosis is that of ovarian remnant syndrome. The presence of erythrocytes indicates that some uterine tissue remains and makes the diagnosis simpler.

ii. Collection of a vaginal smear when the bitch has clinical signs of oestrus provides a simple and rapid method of diagnosis. It is also possible to measure peripheral plasma progesterone concentrations two weeks after the signs of oestrus have disappeared. Raised progesterone concentrations are diagnostic for luteal tissue present within the ovarian remnant. Investigative techniques include diagnostic laparoscopy or laparotomy.

iii. The differential diagnoses for recurrent vulval discharge in an ovariohysterectomized bitch include vaginitis (which may be related to changes in local immunity associated with removal of the ovaries), certain bacterial or viral infections (although these are very rare as primary causes), chemical irritation (e.g. urine), mechanical irritation (foreign bodies), vaginal or urethral neoplasia, stump pyometra and diseases of the urinary tract. Differential diagnoses for attractiveness to males includes vaginitis and anal gland disease.

iv. Surgical removal of the ovarian remnant will be curative. Frequently the remnant is associated with the right ovarian pedicle, and surgery is best performed during or shortly after oestrus when the ovarian tissue reaches its maximum size.

79 i. There is a severe hypokalaemia and mild renal dysfunction. Elevated urea and creatinine in the face of a relatively dilute urine is consistent with primary renal failure. This may develop as a consequence of the hypokalaemia or, more likely, result in hypokalaemia through potassium loss in urine.

ii. Forelimb hypermetria, broad-based hindlimb stance and apparent muscle pain on palpation may also be seen. Smooth and cardiac muscle may be affected resulting in gastric atony, paralytic ileus, reduced cardiac output and cardiac arrhythmias. Metabolic and renal effects include an attenuated response to glucose loading, metabolic acidosis and polyuria/polydipsia (ADH resistance). Hypokalaemia may initiate, perpetuate and exacerbate pre-existing renal disease.

iii. Potassium supplementation is required for all hypokalaemic cats even if clinical signs are not apparent. Potassium chloride is used for intravenous fluid supplementation unless hypophosphataemia is present when potassium phosphate is preferred. Intravenous fluids containing glucose or bicarbonate should be avoided as these can cause hypokalaemia. Overzealous fluid administration can exacerbate hypokalaemia because of volume expansion, dilution and accelerated urinary potassium loss. Potassium gluconate is preferred for oral supplementation.

80 A three-year-old, male 22.5 kg English Bulldog was evaluated for a five-day history of anorexia and depression. He had vomited on one occasion five days previously. Rectal temperature was 40.1°C (104.2°F). During abdominal palpation, pain was consistently exhibited. The clinical pathology results obtained are shown. Urine cytology revealed many red blood cells, 100–110 white blood cells/hpf, 2–5 granular casts/hpf, many bacteria (rods) and plentiful amorphous crystals.

i. What is your diagnosis?
ii. What diagnostic test would you carry out next?
iii. What are the most common organisms associated with bacterial urinary tract infections in dogs?
iv. Is radiography of any value?

Albumin (g/l)	25
ALP (u/l)	268
ALT (u/l)	43
Total protein (g/l)	66
Urea (mmol/l)	6.8
Creatinine (µmol/l)	97
Glucose (mmol/l)	4.3
Sodium (mmol/l)	139
Potassium (mmol/l)	3.8
Calcium (mmol/l)	2.3
Phosphorus (mmol/l)	1.6
PCV (l/l)	0.41
WBCs ($\times 10^9$/l)	32.5
Neutrophils (seg) ($\times 10^9$/l)	27.3
Neutrophils (bands) ($\times 10^9$/l)	1.95
Lymphocytes ($\times 10^9$/l)	1.3
Monocytes ($\times 10^9$/l)	1.95
Platelets ($\times 10^9$/l)	122
Toxic neutrophils present.	
Urinalysis:	
Colour	Yellow
Turbidity	Cloudy
SG	1.025
pH	6.5
Glucose, ketones, bilirubin	Negative
Protein (qualitative)	1+

81 A four-month-old kitten is presented with persistent diarrhoea and poor growth. The result of faecal analysis is shown (**81**).
i. Identify this parasite.
ii. How would you manage this case?

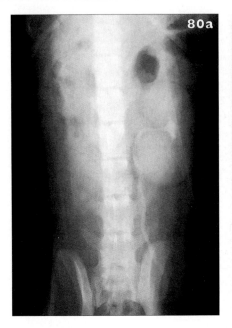
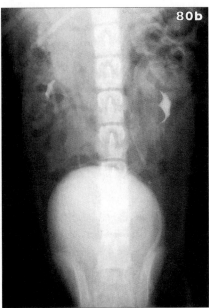

80 i. Pyelonephritis – unilateral with acute sepsis. An active sediment (numerous RBCs, WBCs and casts) is present on urinalysis and an inflammatory process is indicated by the neutrophilia.

ii. Urine culture and sensitivity for aerobic bacteria. The urine sample must be obtained by cystocentesis.

iii. *Escherichia coli, Staphylococcus* spp., *Streptococcus* spp., *Klebsiella* spp., *Proteus* spp.

iv. Excretory urography may be helpful. This relies on excretion of an intravenous contrast material. Any impairment of renal function will reduce the amount of contrast material in the kidney. Urography will tend to rule out other renal abnormalities such as filling defects and renomegaly. Excretory urography was performed in this dog (80a, 80b) and it showed a unilateral reduction in glomerular filtration rate.

81 i. An oocyst of *Isospora felis*.

ii. Infection with *Isospora* is extremely common, particularly in kittens. Although *Isospora* can be a primary pathogen, in the majority of cases a self-limiting infection occurs in the absence of any clinical signs. A heavy infection may occur, in association with overcrowding, poor hygiene and stress, and may result in diarrhoea, vomiting, weight loss or poor growth. Where *Isospora* is identified, it is important to search for other causes of the clinical signs (*Salmonella, Campylobacter, Giardia*, intussusception, etc.) as the coccidia may be an incidental finding. If numerous oocysts are found in the faeces, and no other cause for the clinical signs is apparent, treatment is recommended with trimethoprim/sulphadiazine (30 mg/kg daily) or furazolidone (8 mg/kg daily), both given for 7–10 days.

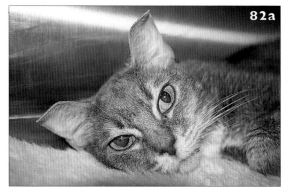

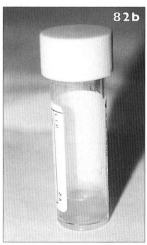

82 A two-year-old, female domestic shorthair cat belonged to a cattery which housed over 15 animals in separate enclosures. They were frequently rotated so that cats were in close contact with one another. This cat was inappetent and lethargic over several days. No other cat was currently ill. This cat had anisocoria with normal pupillary light reactions in the left eye (82a). The right pupil was widely dilated and non-responsive to light. Aqueous flare was present in the right anterior chamber and intraocular pressures were low consistent with uveitis. Chorioretinitis lesions were present on fundic examination. The abdomen was mildly distended with a doughy feel on palpation. Abdominocentesis yielded a thick, viscous yellow fluid (82b). On analysis the fluid was relatively acellular, containing <100 non-degenerate neutrophils, and it had a protein content of 52 g/l. Pertinent laboratory findings included a fasted serum bile acid concentration of 200 µmol/l and a hyperglobulinaemia of 63 g/l with a serum total protein concentration of 92 g//l.

i. What is your presumptive diagnosis?

ii. What further tests could help you make a definitive diagnosis?

iii. What recommendations can you make for the owner of this cattery?

83 A ten-week-old unvaccinated dog, one of a litter of six, died following an acute illness of two days' duration. The pup presented with acute onset depression, vomiting and severe haemorrhagic diarrhoea. The dam was unvaccinated. Piperazine had been prescribed for the pups two weeks previously.

i. What infectious agents would you consider as possible causes of the pup's death?

ii. What advice would you give the breeder?

82 i. In a young, ill cat with anterior uveitis, chorioretinitis, hyperglobulinaemia and a non-septic, viscous, abdominal exudate as depicted in the picture, feline infectious peritonitis (FIP) should be high on your list of differential diagnoses. Other possible causes for the presence of abdominal fluid could include portal hypertension, heart failure and cholangiohepatitis, but these disorders are not usually accompanied by ocular lesions, and such high concentrations of protein in the abdominal fluid with a low cell count is very suspicious of an FIP infection.

ii. Although a coronavirus titre can indicate exposure to the virus that causes FIP, other less virulent coronaviruses may also result in a positive titre. For this reason, this test is considered non-specific and only supportive of a diagnosis if the titre is greatly increased. Animals that are severely ill with active FIP infections may indeed have negative coronavirus titres since the antibodies produced are rapidly bound to the large number of circulating virus particles. This cat had a negative coronavirus titre. The finding of increased gamma immunoglobulins on electrophoresis of the abdominal fluid can also be supportive of a diagnosis of FIP, but the definitive diagnosis is based upon histopathological lesions of perivascular inflammation in affected tissues. On exploratory laparotomy a diffuse, fibrinous debris covered the surface of the liver and other viscera. Histopathology of the liver parenchyma revealed a severe, perivascular granulomatous inflammation consistent with FIP.

iii. Eliminating FIP infection from a cattery can be extremely difficult and frustrating. It is unknown which animals may have been infected with the virus, so it should be assumed that they have all been exposed and the cattery should be kept closed both to the addition of new animals and to the movement of animals to homes with other cats outside of the cattery. The incubation period of FIP infection may be weeks to months or even years. Due to the difficulty in interpreting coronavirus titres, it is neither necessary nor diagnostic to determine titres in these cats. Most cats that are exposed to the virus become resistant to infection and do not become ill. However, a small percentage will become clinically ill with FIP viral-induced disease, and these cats should be quarantined. Treatment of FIP is generally ineffective, and when supportive care fails, euthanasia of ill cats is indicated.

83 i. Canine parvovirus (CPV), canine coronavirus (CCV), salmonellosis, *Clostridium perfringens* or *C. difficile*, *Campylobacter jejuni*, canine distemper virus (CDV).

ii. Submit the pup for a full postmortem examination. Submit rectal swabs (for CPV, CCV and bacterial isolation) and blood (for CPV, CCV and CDV serology) from the other pups. Paired serology can be performed on a second sample taken two weeks later. Vaccinate those pups with a low CPV or CDV antibody titre with a live attenuated CPV or CDV vaccine. Move the pups to an uncontaminated area and use hypochlorite to disinfect the infected environment.

84 A 16-year-old, neutered female domestic shorthair cat presents with acute onset generalized muscle weakness and an inability to lift its head. Although the cat has no history of medical problems, the owners report that she has been losing weight, is polydipsic (drinking out of sinks and bathtubs) and appears to be polyuric. The cat is fed a dry diet and

Urea (mmol/l)	27
Creatinine (µmol/l)	309
Sodium (mmol/l)	145
Potassium (mmol/l)	2.5
Total CO_2 (mmol/l)	8
Calcium (mmol/l)	2.6
Phosphorus (mmol/l)	2.1

there has been no dietary change. Serum biochemistry is performed.

i. What is the likely diagnosis given the cat's age and clinical presentation?
ii. What other diagnostic tests would you perform?
iii. What would be your initial treatment?
iv. What is the prognosis for the generalized muscle weakness?

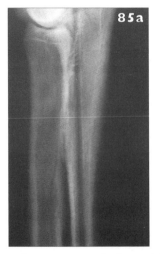

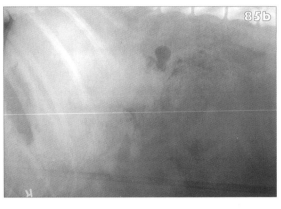

85 A ten-year-old German Shepherd Dog presented with an acute onset stiff gait and reluctance to move. The forelimbs were warm, swollen and painful to digital pressure over the bones. The joints were unremarkable. No pain could be elicited on manipulation of the shoulder, elbow, carpi or metacarpal joints. The owner commented that the dog's abdomen was enlarging and on palpation a large solid mass was found. There were no clinical signs referable to the abdominal or thoracic cavity and thoracic auscultation was unremarkable. Radiography of the forelimb and the abdominal cavity was performed (85a, 85b).

i. What is your interpretation of the radiographs?
ii. What would you recommend to your client?

84 i. The likely cause of the muscle weakness is the hypokalaemia. The polyuria and polydipsia, and raised urea and creatinine values, are consistent with renal failure (probably chronic in nature), which is a cause of hypokalaemia.

ii. Further diagnostic tests should include abdominal radiography to evaluate the entire urinary tract (including renal size), complete urinalysis to investigate the possibility of renal infection, and haematological assessment to determine the presence of anaemia which may develop secondarily to chronic disease or anaemia.

iii. Oral administration of potassium is the safest and preferred route for potassium supplementation as parenteral administration is more likely to result in hyperkalaemia. Parenteral potassium supplementation is reserved for patients that require emergency reversal of hypokalaemia or for patients that cannot or will not accept oral therapy. Potassium gluconate is the salt of choice in cats (2–6 mmol/cat q24h) depending upon the size of the cat and the severity of the hypokalaemia. Potassium citrate is also suitable. Potassium chloride may be administered parenterally at a maintenance dose of 13–20 mmol/l of fluids or, if the cat is hypokalaemic, 20–40 mmol/l of fluids. Do not administer potassium salts at a rate greater than 0.5 mmol/kg/hr.

iv. The prognosis for the generalized muscle weakness is good. It normally resolves within five days of replacement therapy. The prognosis for chronic renal failure is guarded.

85 i. The abdominal radiograph shows a large soft tissue mass in the ventral mid-abdominal region. Small intestinal tissues are displaced dorsally and caudally suggesting that the mass is originating in the cranioventral area of the abdomen and is most likely to be of liver or splenic origin. The diaphragmatic liver lobe is visible cranial to the mass, but neither the caudal liver lobes nor the spleen are visible. The radiographic diagnosis is of neoplasia.

The limb radiograph shows soft tissue swelling and regular periosteal proliferation extending along the length of the radius and ulna. No other bony changes are evident. The radiographic diagnosis is secondary hypertrophic osteopathy (Marie's disease). This is most often associated with thoracic masses, but may develop in association with abdominal masses (neoplasia or infection).

ii. The limb changes are not life-threatening and may resolve to some extent if the mass is removed. Analgesics are indicated. Further diagnostics should be aimed at determining if the mass is benign or malignant. Thoracic radiography is indicated in the first instance to assess for pulmonary metastases. Ultrasonography may be helpful in determining its origin. If this is unavailable, administration of a small amount of barium may be helpful in indicating the position of the stomach, which again may provide some clue as to whether the mass is spleen or liver. Ultimately though, an exploratory laparotomy is required to assess whether removal is feasible or not. In this case the neoplasm was a haemangiosarcoma and euthanasia was performed.

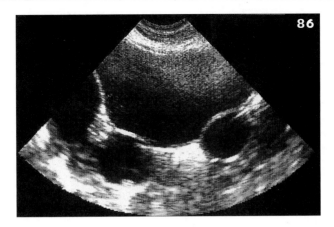

86 A six-year-old, entire bitch has a white mucoid vulval discharge which commenced four weeks after mating. Otherwise she is clinically normal. An ultrasound examination of the caudal abdomen has been performed from the ventral midline (86).
i. What are the ultrasonographic findings, and what is the likely diagnosis?
ii. How might this condition be treated surgically?
iii. How might this condition be treated medically?
iv. What is the likely subsequent fertility?

87 You examine a five-year-old, male Miniature Schnauzer for vomiting of two days' duration. Results of laboratory evaluation are shown.
i. What is your interpretation of the azotaemia: pre-renal, renal or post-renal?
ii. What is your diagnosis?
iii. What are granular casts, and what is their significance?

Urea (mmol/l)	23
Creatinine (μmol/l)	186
Sodium (mmol/l)	147
Potassium (mmol/l)	4.9
Total CO_2 (mmol/l)	17
Calcium (mmol/l)	2.5
Phosphorus (mmol/l)	1.6
Serum amylase (u/l)	7,200
Urine SG	1.047
Urine protein	Negative
Urine casts	Moderate granular

86 i. The image shows a large anechoic bladder close to the abdominal wall. Dorsal to the bladder (ventral in this image) there are three almost circular discrete fluid-filled structures with a diameter of between 2.0 and 2.5 cm. These structures are different sections of the uterus and it would appear that the uterus is enlarged and fluid filled. A definitive diagnosis cannot be made from an image taken in one plane, and a second image at 90° to the first is required. The most likely diagnoses are pyometra and pregnancy, both of which occur at the same time of the oestrous cycle. This case is a pyometra and can be distinguished from a pregnancy by the absence of fetal tissue and membranes. By imaging in a second plane it was demonstrated that the fluid-filled zones were confluent rather than discrete as found during pregnancy. It is common for bitches to have a mucoid vulval discharge during pregnancy, and often they may have a reduced appetite at the time of implantation.

ii. The treatment of choice for bitches with pyometra remains ovariohysterectomy combined with appropriate fluid and antimicrobial therapy. Attempts have been made to drain the uterine fluid using a catheter placed via the cervix. However, this technique is difficult to perform, therefore surgically introduced drains placed transcervically via a hysterotomy have been advocated by some workers. These are used to flush the uterus after surgery. Variable success rates have been described following this surgical technique and generally it is not considered to be a viable therapy.

iii. Medical treatment may be attempted in all cases of pyometra, although this is more appropriate in cases of open cervix pyometra; most regimes use uterine ecbolic agents that may cause uterine rupture if the cervix is closed. Low doses of prostaglandin administered twice daily for up to one week may be successful, although side-effects of prostaglandin therapy (including restlessness, pacing, hypersalivation, tachypnoea, vomiting, diarrhoea, pyrexia, abdominal pain) are common. Prostaglandin therapy should be combined with appropriate broad-spectrum antimicrobial agents and intravenous fluid administration. Prostaglandins are useful since as well as promoting uterine contraction they cause lysis of the corpora lutea and a reduction in plasma progesterone concentrations.

iv. Medical treatment using prostaglandins has achieved success rates of up to 80% with approximately 25% of animals eventually producing litters. However, long-term complications including anoestrus, recurrence of pyometra, failure to conceive and abortion are not uncommon.

87 i. Pre-renal azotaemia because the urine SG is appropriately concentrated with azotaemia.

ii. Pancreatitis with pre-renal azotaemia due to dehydration.

iii. Casts are cylindrical-shaped structures composed of mucoprotein and occasionally cells and cellular debris. Granular casts represent epithelial casts that have disintegrated. Epithelial, fatty, granular and waxy casts are usually associated with degeneration or necrosis of tubular epithelial cells.

88 These ultrasound images are of the abdomen of an 18-week-old German Shepherd Dog with an acute history of lethargy, vomiting and haemorrhagic diarrhoea (88a, 88b). A double-layered tubular structure is visible.

i. What is the most likely diagnosis?

ii. What would you expect to be able to palpate within the abdomen?

iii. How would you confirm the diagnosis?

iv. How would you treat this dog and prevent recurrence?

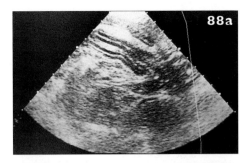

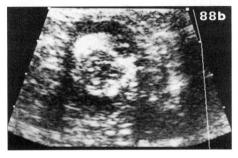

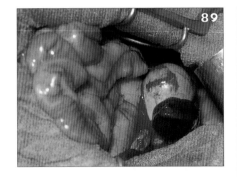

89 An 11-year-old, male Miniature Poodle became inappetent and vomited intermittently for one month. Weight loss and jaundice had developed recently. The laboratory data are shown. Abdominal radiographs were unremarkable. Exploratory laparotomy was performed.

PCV (l/l)	0.47
Hb (g/l)	88
WBCs ($\times 10^9$/l)	26.5
Neutrophils: bands ($\times 10^9$/l)	3.6
Neutrophils: segmented ($\times 10^9$/l)	18.9
Lymphocytes ($\times 10^9$/l)	0.8
Monocytes ($\times 10^9$/l)	3.2
Albumin (g/l)	309
Globulin (g/l)	38
Bilirubin (µmol/l)	83
ALT (u/l)	1,469
ALP (u/l)	2,740
Cholesterol (mmol/l)	10.8
Amylase (u/l)	366

i. What was the reason for performing surgery in this patient?

ii. What comments would you make on the surgical picture (89)?

iii. How would you proceed at surgery?

88 i. The ultrasound image is characteristic of an intussusception.

ii. A cylindrical/sausage-shaped, doughy mass in the mid-abdomen. Faecal material might have a similar feel but should deform with gentle pressure.

iii. Plain and barium contrast radiographs might be helpful in identifying an intussusception. A 'coiled-spring' appearance seen on barium enema can also be helpful. Ileocolic intussusception may protrude through the anus. It can be distinguished from a rectal prolapse by the ability to pass a probe (such as a thermometer) through the anus alongside the intussusceptum. In this case the results of abdominal palpation and ultrasound imaging are sufficient to justify an exploratory laparotomy.

iv. Surgical reduction of the intussusception is attempted at laparotomy, but often the presence of adhesions and bowel necrosis necessitates intestinal resection and end-to-end anastomosis. Postoperatively, feeding of liquid/soft food is reinstituted early in the recovery phase. Prolonged withholding of food is likely to delay healing and increase the risk of wound dehiscence. Attempts to prevent recurrence by giving antimuscarinic agents (e.g. hyoscine [Buscopan Compositum]) do not have a sound physiological basis as they cause ileus, delaying restoration of normal intestinal peristalsis. Enteroplication, by suturing adjacent loops of bowel, is the only guaranteed method of preventing recurrence.

89 i. Jaundice in this dog is hepatic or posthepatic. Haematology shows a neutrophilia with marked left shift (indicative of an inflammatory, possibly infectious process), lymphopenia and monocytosis. Hyperglobulinaemia suggests chronic antigenic stimulation. The dog is hyperbilirubinaemic, which looks predominantly cholestatic (very high ALP), although there is obvious hepatocellular involvement (high ALT). Cholesterol is high, and in a dog with cholestatic jaundice this may point towards extrahepatic biliary obstruction; other differentials are hypothyroidism, diabetes mellitus, hyperadrenocorticism, nephrotic syndrome and hyperlipidaemia. Amylase is normal, which makes pancreatitis as a cause of bile duct compression less likely, although it does not rule it out. The overall impression is of a dog with cholestatic jaundice that may have an inflammatory component; possible causes would be cholangiohepatitis, cholelithiasis and neoplasia. Ultrasound would have been useful to distinguish between intrahepatic or extrahepatic obstruction. If the biliary tree was normal on ultrasonography, percutaneous liver biopsy might have been performed. In this case, ultrasound was not available and the chronic and progressive nature of signs and the possibility of extrahepatic biliary obstruction led to the decision to explore the liver and bile ducts surgically.

ii. The gallbladder looks thickened and moderately distended, suggestive of cholecystitis and partial obstruction.

iii. An attempt should be made to express the gallbladder to see if the bile duct is patent, and to inspect the area surrounding the bile duct for signs of external compression. Bile should be aspirated for culture, and liver biopsies should be obtained for histopathology and culture. In this case, calculi were palpated in the gallbladder and removed via a cholecystotomy. Choleliths are often radiolucent and do not show up on routine radiographs. It is important to culture choleliths as well as bile. In this dog, *Escherichia coli* was cultured from bile and choleliths, and liver biopsies showed suppurative cholangiohepatitis.

90 A two-year-old, neutered male domestic shorthair cat has recently been introduced to a household with seven other cats. Within a few days of acquiring the cat the owner noticed persistent, liquid diarrhoea, although the cat appeared bright and was eating well. The cat has not improved following starvation for 48 hours and introduction of a simple, commercial (chicken and rice based) diet for two weeks, and is presented for further investigation. The cat is shown (90).

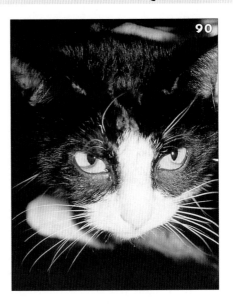

i. What are your differential diagnoses for this cat?
ii. What, if any, further investigations would you suggest?
iii. What advice/prognosis would you give to the owner?

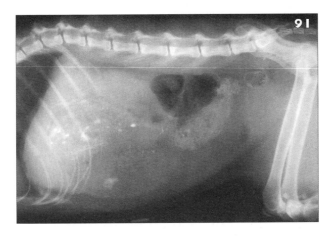

91 A three-year-old crossbreed dog is presented with a history of chronic vomiting of several months' duration and slight weight loss. The vomitus comprises digested food and occurs at variable times after eating ranging from one to several hours. The dog has a good appetite. Serum biochemistry and haematology were unremarkable. An abdominal radiograph was taken (91).
i. What is your interpretation of the radiograph?
ii. What are your main differential diagnoses?
iii. What other diagnostic tests might you consider performing?

90 i. The cat is displaying bilateral protrusion of the third eyelids. The most likely diagnosis in this individual would be the 'prolapsed nictitating membrane/chronic diarrhoea' (PNM/CD) syndrome or Haws syndrome. Other differential diagnoses would include infection with bacterial or parasitic intestinal pathogens (e.g. *Salmonella*, *Campylobacter*, *Giardia*), inflammatory bowel disease, dietary hypersensitivity or intolerance, intestinal neoplasia and partial intestinal obstruction.
ii. If clinical signs are fully compatible with PNM/CD, further investigations may not be indicated, although screening of faecal samples for bacterial pathogens and parasites is sensible.
iii. Most cats affected with PNM/CD remain bright and continue to eat well, and generally there is little or no weight loss despite persistent and often severe small intestinal diarrhoea. The PNM/CD syndrome has been recognized as a clinical entity for many years, although its precise cause remains elusive. Epidemiological evidence strongly supports an infectious, contagious aetiology (probably viral in origin); a torovirus has been suggested, although this has yet to be proven. In view of the contagious nature of the disease, there is a high probability that some, or all, of the other cats in the household will develop the same clinical signs. Provided the cats remain otherwise healthy, and the diarrhoea does not cause a problem to the owner, there is no necessity to treat affected individuals. If treatment is undertaken, antibiotics should be avoided as there is no rationale for their use in this disease. A simple, highly digestible diet may be advised, and can be combined with a faecal bulking agent (e.g. Peridale Granules or Isogel) and/or a motility modifier such as loperamide. In many cases medical intervention makes little difference to the severity of the diarrhoea. Although signs may be protracted, affected cats will eventually recover without developing any apparent long-term consequences.

91 i. The abdominal radiograph shows the stomach to be distended. The pylorus is displaced ventrocaudally. The stomach contains small mineral densities which represent previously ingested material retained in the stomach. This 'gravel' sign and the presence of gastric dilatation, taken with the clinical signs, is strongly suggestive of a gastric outflow problem or gastric hypomotility.
ii. The main differential causes of this dog's problem are intraluminal masses and/or foreign bodies, mucosal or mural proliferative disorders (e.g. gastric antral mucosal hypertrophy, hypertrophic gastritis, pyloric hypertrophy) or compression of the outflow tract by masses or organs outside the stomach or malposition of the stomach.
iii. A barium study may be helpful in documenting impaired gastric outflow. Endoscopy is required to determine the cause of any obstruction. Mucosal biopsies should be taken even if the gross appearance is normal.

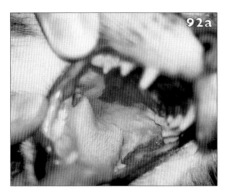
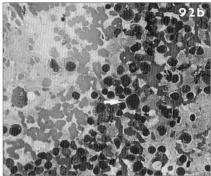

92 A two-year-old, male cat presented with a three-week history of slowly progressive jaundice and lethargy, with a recent onset of vomiting in the last two days. On physical examination the cat was alert and responsive with bright yellow mucous membranes (**92a**), a rough, unkempt hair coat and palpable hepatomegaly. Pertinent laboratory findings on haematological and biochemical profiles included: PCV 0.19 l/l, reticulocyte count 0.3%, ALP 233 u/l, ALT 308 u/l, urea 12 mmol/l, creatinine 212 µmol/l, total bilirubin 123 µmol/l and fasting serum bile acids 89 µmol/l. A fine-needle aspirate of the liver parenchyma was obtained (**92b**).

i. Based on the cytology of the aspirate, what is your diagnosis?
ii. What other test(s) should be performed?
iii. What is the prognosis, and what are the options for treatment?

93 Which of these statements about hyperadrenocorticism (HAC) are true and which are false?

i. Most cases of HAC present acutely with signs such as vomiting, diarrhoea and seizures.
ii. Urinary tract infections are very unusual in dogs with HAC.
iii. Alopecia is expected in all cases of HAC.
iv. Calcification of bronchial walls may be seen radiographically in animals with HAC.
v. Testicular atrophy is common in male dogs with HAC.

92 i. The cells seen on the fine-needle aspirate cytology are a homogeneous population of large, immature lymphoid cells with a low nuclear to cytoplasm ratio consistent with hepatic lymphoma. The arrow is indicating an enlarged, basophilic lymphoblastic cell with malignant characteristics. Multicentric lymphoma in cats can affect one or more organ systems including liver, renal, ocular, spleen and/or deep and superficial lymph nodes. The presence of azotaemia and polydipsia may reflect renal lymphomatous infiltration as well.

ii. Approximately 70% of cats with multicentric lymphoma test positive for FeLV. FeLV infection may be responsible for the non-regenerative anaemia due to the suppressive effects of the virus on the bone marrow. Other helpful diagnostic tests to stage the disease, and determine the extent of organ involvement, might include a renal and bone marrow aspirate and a thoracic radiograph.

iii. Lymphoma is a systemic disease and chemotherapy is the preferred treatment modality. Surgical reduction of tumour mass and/or radiotherapy have been shown to be effective in reducing a large, focal tumour burden, but systemic chemotherapeutic treatment is also usually required. The goal of treatment with chemotherapy is to establish a good, normal quality of life, with minimal side-effects, for six months to one year or more. Several different chemotherapy protocols have proven to be effective; these commonly include drugs such as prednisolone, vincristine, doxorubicin, methotrexate and L-asparaginase. Lymphoma is not a curable disease; important considerations for deciding upon an appropriate treatment regime include time and financial constraints, and the disposition of the patient.

93 i. False. HAC is a chronic, slowly progressive disorder.
ii. False. Urinary tract infections are commonly found in animals with HAC.
iii. False. Alopecia is recognized in most but not all cases of HAC.
iv. True.
v. True.

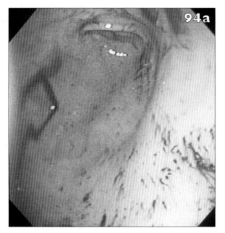 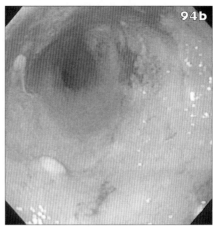

94 A seven-year-old, male Dobermann has chronic diarrhoea with weight loss. He vomits bile and/or fresh blood intermittently and there is evidence of melena on rectal examination. An eosinophilia (5.4×10^9/l) is noted. Gastroscopy reveals numerous paint brush haemorrhages, seen here in the pyloric antrum (**94a**), and evidence that the dog has been eating grass. In the duodenum the mucosa is irregular and friable and haemorrhages easily (**94b**); a normal duodenal papilla is also visible in this picture. Histological examination of multiple pinch biopsies confirms a diagnosis of eosinophilic gastroenteritis.

i. Could this diagnosis have been reached without GI biopsies and, if not, why not?
ii. How would you treat this animal?

95 Differentiating non-regenerative from regenerative anaemia is often of crucial importance in the medical investigation of a case. The morphological features of regeneration are macrocytosis (increased MCV), hypochromia, polychromasia and the presence of nRBCs.

i. Which of these is the most reliable indicator of regeneration?
ii. Which of these is most susceptible to simple artefact?
iii. How can the adequacy of a regenerative response be established objectively?

94 & 95: Answers

94 i. Chronic intermittent vomiting, diarrhoea and weight loss are suggestive of inflammatory bowel disease. GI haemorrhage is commonly seen with eosinophilic infiltrates, and the peripheral eosinophilia is consistent with eosinophilic enteritis. However, eosinophilia is not a consistent finding in eosinophilic gastroenteritis and is not diagnostic. Parasitism, especially in heartworm-endemic areas, is a more common cause of eosinophilia. A definitive diagnosis of eosinophilic gastroenteritis must be made with a biopsy before rational therapy can be prescribed. Luminal parasites, including *Giardia*, could be the causative agent, and visceral larva migrans has also been suggested as a potential cause.

ii. Treatment with fenbendazole (50 mg/kg p/o q24h for 3 days) to eliminate parasites should be initiated prior to immunosuppressive therapy. The eosinophilic mucosal infiltrate may represent a manifestation of a dietary sensitivity and an exclusion diet trial is also indicated. A novel diet containing single protein and carbohydrate sources which the patient is not currently eating are fed as the sole dietary intake. Chicken, catfish, venison, mutton or fish, with rice or potato, are found in some of the available commercial products, although home-cooked diets may be preferred. The trial period is usually three weeks, although if there is partial improvement the trial should be extended for up to ten weeks. Failure to improve with an exclusion diet suggests idiopathic inflammatory bowel disease, and treatment is with immunosuppressive drugs – prednisolone (1–2 mg/kg p/o q12h for 2–4 weeks then tapered off over several months assuming an initial positive response). Failure to respond or development of iatrogenic hyperadrenocorticism indicate a need for more potent immunosuppressive drugs, e.g. azathioprine.

95 i. Polychromasia nearly always indicates regeneration. Subjectively, the amount of polychromasia reflects the adequacy of regeneration. Nucleated RBCs can be present in non-regenerative anaemias involving bone marrow damage. Hypochromia is a feature of iron deficiency anaemias as well as regenerative anaemia. Macrocytes observed in a blood film are quite reliable indicators of regeneration, but the index of cell size, the MCV, is an inaccurate reflection of the degree of macrocytosis.

ii. The MCV cannot be relied upon as an indicator of regeneration. Erythrocyte swelling occurs rapidly in blood samples that are not refrigerated and will occur to an unpredictable degree in samples sent for analysis. The MCV is a calculated parameter which is affected by the calibration of automated analysers. Most analysers are produced for human use but they measure the MCV of canine RBCs reliably. However, due to the small size of feline RBCs, they must be recalibrated. If laboratories analyse a variety of samples, recalibration may not be a practical consideration and consequently feline MCVs may be erroneous.

iii. A reticulocyte count should be performed on blood samples stained with the vital stain methylene blue. Reticulocyte numbers may be interpreted as the actual value, or a reticulocyte production index (RPI) may be calculated.

RPI = (% reticulocytes × patient PCV/normal PCV)/correction factor

Normal PCV values: dog 0.45 l/l; cat 0.35 l/l.

Correction factors: PCV 0.25–0.35 = 1; PCV 0.20–25 = 1.5; PCV 0.15–20 = 2; PCV <0.15 = 2.5.

RPI values >2 suggest adequate regeneration.

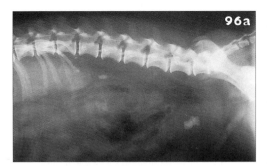

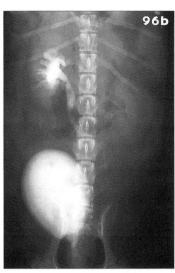

96 A seven-year-old, neutered male Dachshund is presented for evaluation of back pain of less than one day's duration. The previous night he jumped off a chair and has appeared to be in pain since then. Physical examination reveals a tense abdomen and you are able to elicit pain upon palpation of the thoracolumbar region. However, there are no conscious proprioceptive deficits and myotactic reflexes are normal. Thoracolumbar spinal radiography (96a) and excretory urography (96b) is performed.
i. What is your diagnosis?
ii. What is your initial treatment?

97 An eight-year-old, male West Highland White Terrier has mild faecal tenesmus and haemospermia. Rectal examination shows that the prostate gland is enlarged but not painful. The dog is required for breeding. An ultrasound examination of the caudal abdomen has been performed from the ventral midline (97).

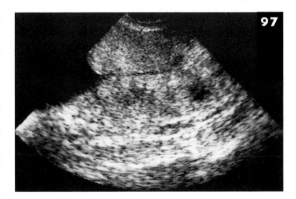

i. What are the ultrasonographic findings, and what is the likely diagnosis?
ii. How can this condition be managed medically?
iii. What effect will medical management have on subsequent fertility?

96 i. Right ureterolith with ureteral obstruction and mild hydronephrosis. The left kidney is structurally normal. Uroliths are present in the bladder. The irregular shape and radiodense appearance is consistent with calcium oxalate. Struvite is also radiodense, but ammonium urate and cystine are only marginally radiodense or are radiolucent.
ii. Because there is ureteral obstruction but the right kidney is functional, the ureterolith should be removed and the right kidney saved if at all possible. The ureterolith was retropulsed into the right renal pelvis and a pyelotomy performed. The dog also had a urocystolith which was removed through a cystotomy.

97 i. The anechoic urinary bladder is present on the left of the ultrasound image. The prostate gland is enlarged bilaterally and the linear anechoic urethra can be seen between the two lobes. The prostatic parenchyma is fairly homogeneous in appearance, although there is a slight increase in the echogenicity. The prostate is a normal shape and has a smooth outline. A one centimetre diameter fluid-filled structure can be identified within the lower lobe. Ultrasonographically the features are of prostatomegaly with a small isolated intraprostatic cyst which are characteristic of benign prostatic hyperplasia. Prostatitis and neoplasia generally produce marked changes in the parenchymal echotexture and the outline of the gland.
ii. Benign prostatic hyperplasia is stimulated by dihydrotestosterone which is irreversibly converted from testosterone by 5-alpha-reductase within the prostate. Castration is a relatively simple procedure that removes the source of testosterone and is therefore a suitable treatment. However, in animals that are required for breeding the suppression of testosterone secretion using exogenous progestogens or oestrogens may be temporarily efficacious. These agents should be used with care since both will have a negative feedback effect upon the hypothalamic–pituitary axis, resulting in suppression of spermatogenesis. Additionally, oestrogens may cause prostatic metaplasia. Finasteride is a specific 5-alpha-reductase inhibitor which prevents the conversion of testosterone into dihydrotestosterone. Use of this agent produces a dramatic reduction in the size of the prostate gland and resolution of the clinical signs. It reduces the ejaculate volume, although total sperm output and spermatozoal morphology are unaffected.
iii. Low doses of progestogens may be used infrequently without producing a reduction in fertility. However, repeated administration of high doses causes a reduction in spermatozoal morphology, motility and spermatozoal output, and a subsequent decline in fertility. Despite the marked changes in semen volume produced by finasteride, fertility is maintained for treatments of up to three months duration.

98 A five-year-old Retriever presented with acute onset right hindlimb lameness (7/10 lame). A warm and painful soft tissue swelling was present over the dorsal aspect of the pelvis, extending down the thigh. The dog was pyrexic, depressed and anorectic. Radiographs were taken of the swollen area (**98**). Cytological examination of a fine-needle aspirate from the area showed numerous degenerate and non-degenerate neutrophils, and necrotic cells of unidentifiable morphology. A Gram stain of the aspirate demonstrated many short, fat gram-positive rods with few oval subterminal spores. Chains of bacteria were present.

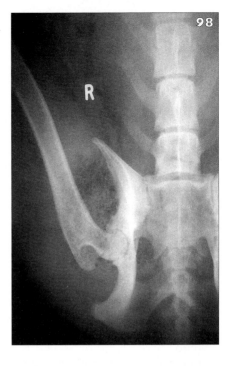

i. What is your diagnosis?
ii. How might you confirm your diagnosis?
iii. What treatment would you recommend?
iv. What other disorders may other species of this bacteria cause?

99 This is an endoscopic view of the pyloric antrum of a three-year-old Cocker Spaniel, recently released from quarantine, who has been violently retching and vomiting three times daily for three weeks (**99**).
i. Can you spot the cause of this dog's problems?
ii. What is the therapy?

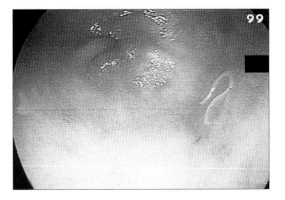

98 i. On the radiograph there is a large radiolucent diffuse gas shadow within the tissues lateral to the pelvis. The cytology is consistent with inflammation and necrosis. The bacteria on the Gram stain were identified morphologically as a *Clostridium* spp., possibly *C. perfringens*. The presumptive diagnosis was gas gangrene.

ii. Histopathology may be helpful. Bacteriology is essential. *C. perfringens* is an anaerobic organism and precautions must be taken to ensure that the bacteria does not die before plating out, i.e. samples should be exposed to air for the minimum time possible.

iii. Clostridial organisms are very sensitive to penicillins and to metronidazole. Treatment with intravenous antibiotics is indicated. The abscessated area should be surgically explored and necrotic tissue removed. The area may be cleansed with dilute hydrogen peroxide which, as it degrades, releases oxygen, thereby killing the bacterium.

iv. Clostridial organisms may be associated with a variety of diseases:

• *C. perfringens* is often isolated from faecal samples and is considered a normal enteric commensal. On occasions it is thought that *C. difficile* and *C. perfringens* may be responsible for severe haemorrhagic diarrhoea, or colitis.

• Enterotoxaemia due to clostridia is rare in dogs and cats, but may occur as an extension of a *C. perfringens* enteric infection.

• Infection with neurotropic clostridia, e.g. *C. tetani* and *C. botulinum*, do occur, with tetanus being more common. These organisms are non-invasive and cause disease through their production of neurotoxins.

• Histotoxic clostridial infections are very rare but should be considered in any case where there is extensive soft tissue necrosis/damage. They most often develop following trauma where bruising and soft tissue damage has resulted in tissues becoming hypoxic, thereby allowing dormant spores to grow.

99 i. A single, white gastric nematode is visible to the lower right of the pyloric sphincter. The remaining gastric mucosa in this area appears grossly normal. This worm was identified as belonging to the genus *Physaloptera*. Although infrequent, dogs and cats may serve as natural hosts for *Physaloptera* and acquire infection via ingesting cockroaches, crickets or beetles which serve as intermediate hosts. Once mature, the parasites reside in the mucosa of the proximal GI tract, creating inflammatory lesions and vomiting.

ii. Routine deworming is important in any pet, and the findings in this dog underscore the need for ruling out the simple options prior to embarking on expensive diagnostics. Pyrantel (5 mg/kg p/o repeated in 7 days) or fenbendazole (50 mg/kg p/o q24h for 3 consecutive days repeated in 3 weeks) should rid the dog of this parasite.

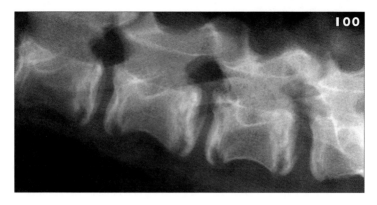

100 This radiograph (100) was taken from a 12-month-old dog of small stature.
i. What is your diagnosis?
ii. What hormonal abnormality is associated with this condition?

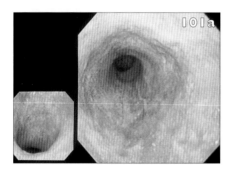

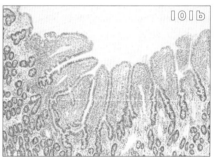

101 An eight-year-old, female Golden Retriever is presented for repeated episodes of vomiting bile, and watery diarrhoea. Episodes have been occurring for over a year, initially only every three to four weeks, but recently they have become more frequent and more severe. In addition, the appetite has decreased, weight loss has occurred and between episodes the dog appears lethargic. A minimum data base of haematology, serum biochemistry, urinalysis, faecal parasitology and bacteriology and abdominal radiography is unhelpful. Serum folate is normal but cobalamin (24 ng/l) is markedly decreased. Endoscopy is performed and the intestinal mucosa is very irregular and friable (101a). Duodenal juice culture is normal (<10^3 cfu/ml). Histological examination of pinch biopsy specimens reveals shortening and distortion of villi and infiltration of the lamina propria with lymphocytes and plasma cells (101b).
i. What is the diagnosis in this case?
ii. What is the treatment?

100 i. Epiphyseal dysgenesis. There is delayed closure of the physes which have an irregular moth-eaten appearance classical of epiphyseal dysgenesis.
ii. Congenital hypothyroidism. Delayed or stunted growth with epiphyseal dysgenesis are the hallmarks of congenital hypothyroidism. Other clinical signs which may be seen are similar to those exhibited in adult-onset hypothyroidism. Goitre may also be a feature depending on the underlying cause of the hypothyroidism.

101 i. The history is typical of IBD, a collective term for various histological descriptions of intestinal mucosal inflammation. In this case the condition would be lymphocytic-plasmacytic enteritis (LPE) because of the predominant cell type present. This is the commonest form of IBD in dogs and is usually idiopathic, although it may develop in response to luminal antigens (bacteria or food). Despite the reduction in serum cobalamin, which might indicate SIBO, quantitative duodenal juice culture did not confirm the diagnosis; the reduction in cobalamin is most likely the result of inflammatory infiltration of the ileum where cobalamin is absorbed.
ii. Antibiotics are not usually indicated in LPE, although they are frequently given as idiopathic LPE is routinely treated with immunosuppressive drugs, and secondary SIBO may exist. Metronidazole (10–20 mg/kg p/o q8–12h) is sometimes used not only for its antibacterial action but because it also modulates cell-mediated immune responses. The immunosuppressive drug of first choice is prednisolone (1–2 mg/kg p/o q12h for up to 4 weeks) until signs are controlled. The dosage is reduced over several months until all medication is stopped or the minimum controlling dose is identified: 5–10 mg q48h would be acceptable. If prednisolone alone does not provide control or if severe iatrogenic hyperadrenocorticism develops, immunosuppression can be enhanced with azathioprine (2 mg/kg p/o q24h for 1–2 weeks, reducing to alternate day therapy with the prednisolone). Azathioprine has potentially disastrous side-effects (e.g. bone marrow suppression) and is not safe without histological evidence of LPE. A positive response to an exclusion diet would suggest a dietary sensitivity. A novel diet containing single protein and carbohydrate sources is fed as the sole dietary intake for three weeks. Chicken, catfish, venison, mutton or fish, with rice or potato, are preferred. If there is improvement, the trial should be extended for up to ten weeks. A strict exclusion diet will only be beneficial if the changes are a manifestation of a dietary sensitivity, but feeding any hypoallergenic diet (i.e. easily digested and low antigenic diversity) may be helpful whenever digestive capacity is impaired. As cobalamin malabsorption is present, parenteral administration (250–500 µg/dog monthly) is indicated. General vitamin-mineral supplementation may be worthwhile.

102 A young farm dog presents with pallor and tachypnoea. The farmer reports having put down some rat baits three days earlier. He thinks it is unlikely that the dog had access to them. The in-house haematological profile and a photomicrograph of the blood smear (**102**) are shown.

WBCs (× 10⁹/l)	23.2
PCV (l/l)	0.21
Granulocytes (× 10⁹/l)	17.4 (75%)
Lymphocytes/ monocytes (× 10⁹/l)	5.8 (25%)
Platelets (× 10⁹/l)	110

i. Is the anaemia regenerative or non-regenerative?

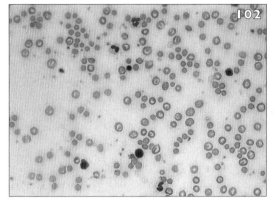

The dog urinates grossly blood-stained urine in the surgery and you send off a sodium citrate sample for urgent measurement of the coagulation times. You treat the dog with vitamin K1. The prothrombin time (PT) is 30 seconds and the activated partial thromboplastin time (APTT) is 25 seconds.

ii. Is vitamin K1 likely to be the correct therapeutic agent in this case? If the answer is yes, why?

iii. What other critical information should be obtained from the farmer?

103 This squash preparation was made from a gastric mucosal biopsy taken from a chronically vomiting dog (**103**).

i. What is the white arrow indicating?

ii. What significance might this have in this dog?

iii. Assuming no other significant lesions or causes of the vomiting are found, how should this dog be treated?

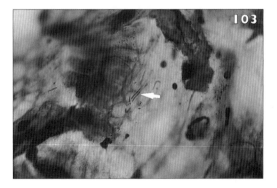

102 i. This is a regenerative anaemia showing polychromasia, anisocytosis, nRBCs and a mildly low platelet count.

ii. Most cases of anticoagulant toxicosis begin to show intensified bleeding symptoms three days after ingestion. At this time the PT will be markedly prolonged due to the short half-life of factor VII and the APTT will be mildly to moderately prolonged due to the longer half-lives of factors IX and X. This profile would therefore be typical of anticoagulant toxicosis of three days' duration, and vitamin K1 would be the therapeutic agent of choice.

iii. It is very important to establish which anticoagulant rodenticide was present in the bait. In this case the farmer reported that it was difacinone. This is a second generation rodenticide with a long half-life and will require vitamin K1 therapy for a period of at least one month. Had the anticoagulant been warfarin, the anticipated duration of therapy would be one week.

103 i. Two parallel, long, thin spiral organisms within the background matrix of cellular debris. These spirochaetes within the stomach are most commonly *Helicobacter* spp. They survive within the acidic environment of the stomach by producing the enzyme urease and surrounding themselves with a protective alkaline layer.

ii. In humans the presence of *Helicobacter* infections is strongly correlated with chronic gastritis, gastric and duodenal ulcers, and gastric neoplasia such as carcinoma and lymphoma. In veterinary medicine, *Helicobacter* spp. have been isolated from both normal dogs and cats and in diseased animals; however, there is no increased prevalence in either population. At this time, many studies are in progress to investigate the role of these organisms in canine and feline gastric disease, but there is no evidence to suggest that *Helicobacter* infection is an important factor in the development of gastritis or gastric ulcers in dogs and cats.

iii. If no underlying organic disease is found on investigation, dietary management should perhaps be attempted initially to rule out dietary intolerances or food hypersensitivities. The decision to treat for *Helicobacter* infection should reflect the degree of inflammation seen on mucosal histopathology in response to the presence of the organisms; the success of this therapy should be determined by the improvement in histological lesions and eradication of the organism. Triple therapy with amoxycillin (10 mg/kg p/o q8h), metronidazole (4 mg/kg p/o q8h) and bismuth subcitrate (1–2 mg/kg p/o q8h) may be used for 14 days. Additional therapy with cimetidine (5–10 mg/kg p/o q8h) or omeprazole (2 mg/kg q24h) has been thought to be effective as well.

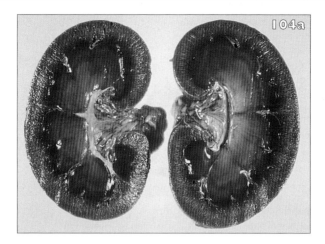

104 A kidney from a three-year-old, male Labrador that died of acute renal failure is shown (**104a**).
i. What is your diagnosis?
ii. What test(s) can be used to confirm this diagnosis?
iii. If the dog had been examined within eight hours of ingestion of the toxin, what drugs may have been used as treatment?

105 A five-year-old, male Labrador is presented with sudden onset pain and swelling of the left scrotum of 12 hours' duration. The swelling extends from the external inguinal ring to the ventral scrotum, and the scrotal skin has been severely self-traumatized. A unilateral castration was performed (**105**).
i. What are the features of the removed tissue, and what is the likely diagnosis?
ii. What differential diagnoses are there for this condition?
iii. How may the condition be accurately diagnosed?
iv. What treatment options are available?

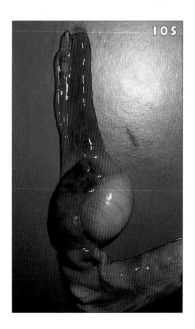

104 i. Ethylene glycol toxicity resulting in acute renal failure. The grit is calcium oxalate crystals that are obstructing the renal tubules. The crystals are shown in **104b**.

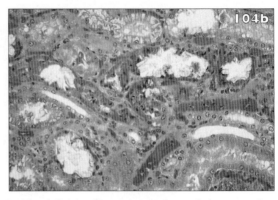

ii. The diagnosis can be supported by finding a high anion gap metabolic acidosis, presence of calcium oxalate crystals in urine sediment, azotaemia with inappropriately low urine SG (renal failure), hypocalcaemia and hypoglycaemia. The definitive diagnosis may be made by measuring ethylene glycol concentrations in blood.

iii. In addition to supportive care and gastric lavage with activated charcoal, preventing metabolism of ethylene glycol by hepatic alcohol dehydrogenase should be attempted. The most effective inhibitor of alcohol dehydrogenase activity is 4-methylpyrazole (4-MP) which does not cause CNS depression. The recommended dose is 20 mg/kg i/v of a 5% solution initially followed by 15 mg/kg i/v at 12 and 24 hours and 5 mg/kg i/v at 36 hours. Ethanol has a higher affinity for alcohol dehydrogenase than does ethylene glycol and this may be used to compete for the enzyme; CNS depression is common with ethanol (5.5 ml/kg i/v of 20% ethanol q4h for 5 treatments, and then q6h on 4 more occasions).

105 i. There is marked swelling and haemorrhage of the spermatic cord, ductus deferens and epididymis. There has been rotation of the spermatic cord and testis around the vertical axis followed by swelling of the associated tissues. The condition is called torsion of the spermatic cord, although it is sometimes referred to as testicular torsion.

ii. The aetiology of torsion of the spermatic cord is unknown, although it may be related to rupture of the scrotal ligament. Conditions that produce similar clinical findings are severe bacterial epididymitis and orchitis (rare in countries in which *Brucella canis* is absent), testicular and scrotal trauma, strangulation of an inguinal hernia and possibly infected or necrotic testicular tumours (although these do not present with sudden onset pain and swelling).

iii. Torsion can be diagnosed most easily on the basis of the clinical signs. Palpation demonstrates the focus of the pain and that the swelling is within the spermatic cord. The lesion is usually unilateral. Scrotal ultrasonography may be useful when there is severe scrotal swelling and may allow the differentiation of torsion from a strangulated hernia.

iv. Prompt surgical removal of the affected testis is essential. Delay in treatment may cause irreversible changes within the adjacent testis due to a rise in temperature. Untreated animals rapidly become systemically unwell.

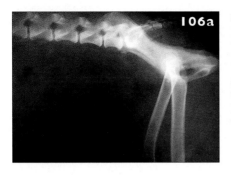

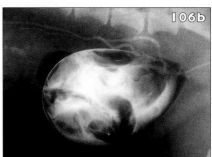

106 A four-year-old Dobermann presented with gross haematuria and difficulty in urinating of four days' duration. The dog was depressed and inappetent. Rectal examination was unremarkable; the prostate was not palpable. Radiography of the lower urinary tract was performed (**106a, 106b**). Clinical biochemistry and haematology values are shown.

i. How would you interpret the radiographs?
ii. What is your interpretation of the blood results?
iii. What is your diagnosis?

Albumin (g/l)	31
Globulin (g/l)	59
Urea (mmol/l)	23.3
Creatinine (μmol/l)	250
ALP (u/l)	950
RBCs ($\times 10^{12}$/l)	4.7
Hb (g/l)	12.6
PCV (l/l)	0.34
MCV (fl)	82
WBCs ($\times 10^9$/l)	33.2
Neut (seg) ($\times 10^9$/l)	22.2
Neut (bands) ($\times 10^9$/l)	7.3
Lymphocytes ($\times 10^9$/l)	3.0
Monocytes ($\times 10^9$/l)	0.7

107 Which of these statements about hyperadrenocorticism (HAC) are true and which are false?
i. The low urine SG seen in animals with HAC develops because cortisol antagonizes antidiuretic hormone (ADH) action and blocks ADH release.
ii. Pulmonary thromboembolism is a potential complication in cases of HAC.
iii. Struvite urolithiasis is common in animals with HAC.
iv. Ketoconazole can be used medically to manage dogs with HAC.
v. Cortisol levels in animals with a pituitary-dependent HAC do not change following administration of ACTH.

108 List the congenital or familial renal diseases associated with the following breeds:
Abyssinian cat; Basenji; Beagle; Bulldog; Cairn Terrier; German Shepherd Dog; Himalayan cat; Irish Wolfhound; Lhasa Apso and Shih Tzu; Norwegian Elkhound; Soft-coated Wheaten Terrier.

106 i. The plain radiograph shows an enlarged prostate and a small bladder. There is no indication of any bony reaction on the vertebrae or pelvis. No sublumbar lymphadenopathy is present and the abdominal organs are normally placed. The lower urinary tract contrast study shows smooth curvilinear filling defects within the bladder. The normal ureters are outlined as a consequence of the earlier administration of intravenous contrast material. A urethral catheter is seen. The filling defects are consistent with blood clots.

ii. There is a marked neutrophilia with a left shift consistent with an inflammatory response, and a mild anaemia which may be due to blood loss. There is a moderate elevation in urea and creatinine consistent with pre-renal azotaemia, primary renal failure or postrenal renal failure. The elevated ALP is consistent with cholestasis, which may reflect the presence of an intrahepatic lesion or extrahepatic inflammation. The elevated globulin reflects the inflammatory process.

iii. Given the prostatomegaly and the degree of dysuria, a prostatic disorder was considered, probably prostatitis or prostatic abscessation.

107 i. True.
ii. True.
iii. False. Calcium oxalate uroliths are more likely to develop because cortisol promotes calcium excretion.
iv. True.
v. False. Cortisol levels should rise dramatically following ACTH administration in animals with pituitary-dependent HAC because adrenal hyperplasia is present. Dogs with adrenal tumours may not show a dramatic rise in cortisol.

108

Breed	Diseases
Abyssinian cat	Amyloidosis
Basenji	Fanconi-like syndrome
Beagle	Unilateral renal agenesis, renal dysplasia, polycystic kidneys
Bulldog	Renal dysplasia
Cairn Terrier	Polycystic kidneys
German Shepherd Dog	Renal cystadenocarcinoma
Himalayan cat	Unilateral renal agenesis, polycystic kidney disease
Irish Wolfhound	Renal dysplasia
Lhasa Apso and Shih Tzu	Renal dysplasia
Norwegian Elkhound	Tubulo-interstitial nephropathy, Fanconi-like syndrome, renal glycosuria
Soft-coated Wheaten Terrier	Renal dysplasia

109 A five-year-old Labrador was mated five weeks previously. One week ago an ultrasound examination demonstrated eight conceptuses; this week seven conceptuses were present. At laparotomy a small conceptus was present between two normal sized swellings (**109**).

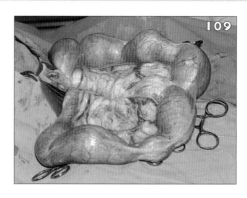

i. What condition is this bitch suffering from, and what is the aetiology of the condition?

ii. What medication might be useful in this case?

iii. Which infective agents can cause resorption and abortion in bitches?

110 A middle-aged German Shepherd Dog presents with a two-week history of progressive lethargy, inappetence and depression. Physical examination is unremarkable except for palpable hepatosplenomegaly and a mild pyrexia. Haematology, serum biochemistry and urinalysis are performed. While examining the tail of the blood film you come across the nucleated cell in the centre of this illustration (**110**).

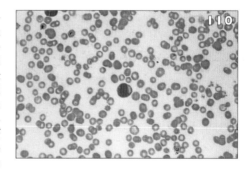

i. Identify the cell.

ii. What is its significance?

The full haematological profile is shown.

iii. How would you interpret these findings?

iv. What is the diagnosis?

RBCs ($\times 10^{12}$/l)	3.09
Hb (g/l)	78
PCV (l/l)	0.26
MCV (fl)	85
MCHC (g/l)	300
nRBCs	0
WBCs ($\times 10^9$/l)	11.1
Neutrophils ($\times 10^9$/l)	0.56
Lymphocytes ($\times 10^9$/l)	5.33
Monocytes ($\times 10^9$/l)	4.11
Eosinophils ($\times 10^9$/l)	0
Basophils ($\times 10^9$/l)	0
Others ($\times 10^9$/l)	1.11

Comment: lymphoblasts 10%; atypical monocytes +++; platelets appear low in the film.

109 i. The bitch has a single isolated resorption. This condition is common in bitches and between five and ten percent of pregnancies suffer isolated resorption without interference with the remaining conceptuses. Bitches are not normally ill and show no clinical signs during the resorption. The condition is not associated with infectious agents and is probably due to competition for uterine space or the failure of an abnormal conceptus. Isolated embryonic resorption can be most reliably diagnosed using real-time B-mode ultrasound where the common features are reduced volume and changes in echogenicity of the embryonic fluid, loss of the heart beat and subsequently the embryonic mass, collapse of the conceptual sac with thickening and inward bulging of the uterine wall, and reduced size in comparison with adjacent conceptuses.
ii. The condition does not require treatment. Many clinicians wrongly attribute embryonic resorption to low plasma progesterone concentrations. Measurement of peripheral progesterone concentrations in these bitches demonstrates that values are within the normal range. Progesterone or progestagen supplementation is not warranted and may prevent or delay parturition (resulting in oversized or dead fetuses respectively) and cause masculinization of female pups and cryptorchidism in male pups.
iii. Embryonic resorption and fetal abortion may have many causes including fetal defects, abnormal maternal environment, infectious agents and trauma. Infectious agents are a relatively rare cause of resorption in the bitch. *Brucella canis* can cause early embryonic death or abortion late in pregnancy followed by a vaginal discharge (this agent is not present in the UK). Other specific infectious causes of abortion include canine distemper virus, canine herpesvirus and *Toxoplasma gondii* infection. In each case the bitch is usually systemically ill and has a vaginal discharge. Fetal death can be confirmed using real-time ultrasonography; loss of fetal fluid and absence of heart beats are noted.

110 i. A lymphoblast. Note the four prominent variably sized nucleoli and the low nuclear/cytoplasmic ratio.
ii. The presence of this cell in the peripheral circulation is abnormal. It is highly suggestive of a lymphoid malignancy.
iii. This is pancytopenia. Normal cell lines are all suppressed with a particularly low neutrophil count. This implies bone marrow disease. The presence of greater than 2% lymphoblasts confirms the presence of a lymphoid malignancy.
iv. Stage V malignant lymphoma.

111 This cat presented because of extreme muscle weakness, forelimb hypermetria, broad-based hindlimb stance, apparent muscle pain on palpation and ventroflexion of the neck (111).

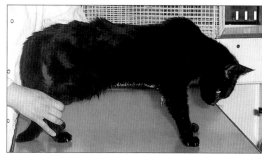

i. Which electrolyte abnormality is most likely to be responsible?
ii. What underlying disease is most likely to result in the above?
iii. In which breed does this disturbance have an inherited predisposition?

112 A poorly grown, five-year-old Golden Retriever presents with ascites and severe depression. There is a marked elevation of ALT and fasting bile acids, a moderate elevation of SAP and low urea and albumin. The ascitic fluid is a transudate. The haematological profile is shown. A photomicrograph taken from the blood smear is shown (112).
i. Comment on the RBC morphology.
ii. How would you interpret this haematology profile?
iii. What diagnosis can be strongly suspected based on the combination of haematology and biochemistry results?

RBCs ($\times 10^{12}$/l)	4.42
Hb (g/l)	40
PCV (l/l)	0.17
MCV (fl)	38
MCHC (g/l)	240
nRBCs	0%
WBCs ($\times 10^9$/l)	17.9
Neutrophils (seg) ($\times 10^9$/l)	14.3
Neutrophils (bands) ($\times 10^9$/l)	2.33
Lymphocytes ($\times 10^9$/l)	0.36
Monocytes ($\times 10^9$/l)	0.54
Eosinophils ($\times 10^9$/l)	0.36

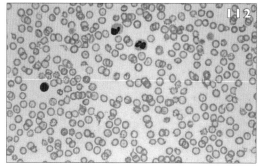

111 i. Hypokalaemia. Clinical signs of hypokalaemia usually become apparent once serum potassium concentrations fall below 3 mmol/l. The most characteristic feature in this cat is ventroflexion of the neck. This clinical picture has often been confused with thiamine deficiency. Elevations in serum creatine kinase concentrations are common.

ii. Chronic renal failure. Potassium concentrations are closely regulated and depend on dietary intake and renal excretion. Disturbances in either can result in hypokalaemia, with chronic renal failure being the most common cause. Potassium loss in the face of renal disease appears to be a peculiar phenomenon of cats. Hypokalaemia can also result from a disturbance in the transcellular shift of potassium, such that total body stores are unchanged; it occurs in metabolic acidosis and following insulin administration.

iii. Burmese. Episodic hypokalaemia has been recognized in related Burmese kittens. Clinical signs appear around 3–4 months of age, are of variable severity and are transient but recurrent in nature. Several weeks may elapse between episodes. The signs are precipitated by stress or exercise and are thought to be due to a sudden shift of potassium from the extracellular to the intracellular compartment.

112 i. The RBCs are markedly microcytic and hypochromic.

ii. This is a severe anaemia which is highly microcytic and hypochromic. There is also a neutrophilia with a left shift suggesting an infectious or inflammatory process. There is a lymphopenia.

iii. The combination of severe hypoalbuminaemia, low urea, markedly elevated fasting bile acids and liver enzyme elevations, with a microcytic, hypochromic anaemia, is quite typical of dogs with portosystemic shunts or chronic hepatopathies. The defect causing the anaemia is a poorly understood abnormality of iron metabolism associated with severe hepatic insufficiency. Portosystemic shunts do not often present with ascites because portal pressure is not usually elevated. This case was a long-standing shunt and the abdominal transudate was probably due to the hypoalbuminaemia (11 g/l) and perhaps a mild elevation in portal pressure.

113 This radiograph is of a neutered male cat with a history of chronic haematuria and dysuria (113). Cytologically, numerous RBCs and calcium oxalate crystals, moderate numbers of inflammatory cells and a few morphologically normal epithelial cells were recognized in a urine sample collected by cystocentesis; no neoplastic cells were seen. Urine pH was 6.5. Gram-negative rods were

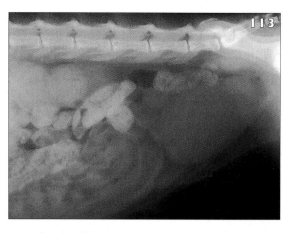

present. Haemolytic colonies were isolated and the organism was a strong lactose fermenter on MacConkey agar. Biochemically the bacteria were indole and methyl red positive, and citrate and Voges-Proskauer negative.

i. Is this radiograph helpful in determining the cause of the haematuria?
ii. How significant are the cytological and bacteriology results?
iii. How common is calcium oxalate urolithiasis in the cat?
iv. How would you manage a cat with calcium oxalate urolithiasis?

114 A two-year-old, female Springer Spaniel has swelling of all mammary glands and the production of a small volume of milk six weeks after her previous oestrus (114).

i. What is the clinical significance of this finding, and what hormonal changes are responsible?
ii. What clinical signs may be associated with this condition in the bitch, and how may they be controlled?

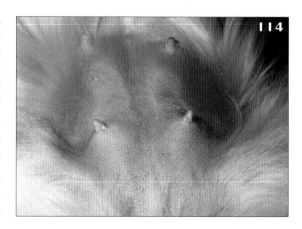

iii. What relationship does this condition have to fertility?

113 i. Plain radiography alone is often not helpful. Large radiopaque calculi may be seen; smaller calculi and radiolucent ones will be missed. Soft tissue causes of haematuria, e.g. polyps and neoplasia, will not be recognized in this radiograph.

ii. The cytology supports the diagnosis of an inflammatory disorder. Calcium oxalate crystals are commonly seen in urine samples. Their presence should alert you to the possibility of urolithiasis. Significantly, the bacteria isolated was *Escherichia coli*.

iii. Calcium oxalate uroliths comprise 27% of all feline uroliths.

iv. Antibiotic therapy is required to manage *E. coli* infection. Existing uroliths should be removed surgically; dietary dissolution is not possible. To prevent recurrence a diet containing reduced concentrations of protein, calcium and sodium that does not promote an acid urine is required. Avoid increased intakes of vitamins C and D. If there is a hypercalcaemia, this should addressed. Potassium citrate may be used to alkalinize urine, thus retarding crystallization of calcium salts, although it predisposes to struvite urolithiasis.

114 i. After oestrus, plasma progesterone concentrations rise and as a consequence, mammary size increases in pregnant and non-pregnant bitches. Corpora lutea produce progesterone for similar periods of time in pregnancy and non-pregnancy. Towards the end of the luteal phase progesterone concentrations fall. At this time prolactin is released from the pituitary gland. This is a luteotropic agent secreted by all bitches that stimulates milk production and some behavioural changes. Mammary development and the secretion of milk should be expected in pregnant and non-pregnant bitches.

ii. Non-pregnant bitches that have mammary swelling and lactation may also have behavioural changes including anorexia, nest making, nursing of inanimate objects and aggression. The hormonal changes that produce these signs occur in all non-pregnant bitches, therefore all non-pregnant bitches can be considered to be pseudopregnant (although the extent to which they demonstrate behavioural changes varies from one individual to the next). In most cases the clinical signs and behavioural changes do not warrant treatment; in some cases the signs may be excessive or may not be tolerated by the owner. In mild cases the administration of diuretic and sedative agents may be useful. If further treatment is necessary, pregnancy and pyometra must be eliminated as differential diagnoses before administration of exogenous reproductive steroids. Progestogens, androgens, oestrogens and combinations of these may be used for treatment. Long treatment periods may be required for complete remission, and it is frequently necessary to use reducing dose regimes to prevent recurrence. The use of dopamine agonists (bromocriptine, cabergoline), which produce a rapid and prolonged inhibition of prolactin secretion, may be used in persistent cases.

iii. There is no relationship between the occurrence of pseudopregnancy and infertility or the subsequent development of cystic endometrial hyperplasia and pyometra.

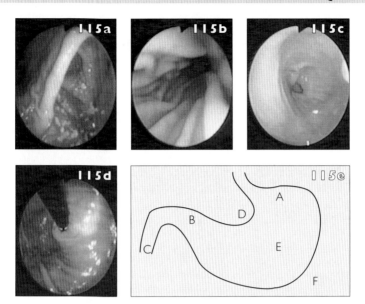

115 Match the letter in the diagram with the appropriate region and endoscopic view that it represents (a view is not included for the greater curvature of the stomach or duodenum).

Region	Endoscopic views
Duodenum	Lesser curvature; angularis (115a)
Lesser curvature	Fundus with rugal folds (115b)
Cardia	Pyloric antrum (115c)
Pyloric antrum	Cardia; scope is retroflexed (115d)
Greater curvature	
Fundus	

116 A nine-month-old, female German Shepherd Dog has suffered intermittent diarrhoea since weaning and has become stunted (116). She has a ravenous appetite and is coprophagic. The most likely diagnosis is idiopathic small intestinal bacterial overgrowth (SIBO).

What tests are available for making a diagnosis of SIBO, and what problems are associated with them?

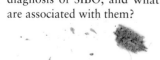

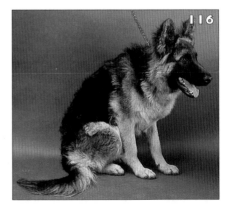

115 A – Cardia (**115d**).
B – Pyloric antrum (**115c**).
C – Duodenum; no matching picture.
D – Lesser curvature (**115a**).
E – Fundus (**115b**).
F – Greater curvature; no matching picture.

116 A diagnosis of idiopathic SIBO is made after ruling out underlying disease. Haematology, biochemistry and urinalysis are used to rule out systemic disease. A faecal examination for parasites such as *Giardia* and a serum TLI for exocrine pancreatic insufficiency should also be performed. Faecal culture does NOT reflect bacterial numbers in the small intestine but is used to rule out *Campylobacter* or chronic salmonellosis. Imaging for an anatomical defect (mass, obstruction, etc.) is indicated. Specific tests include:
• Culture of duodenal juice. The gold standard for the diagnosis of SIBO is quantitative aerobic and anaerobic culture of duodenal juice. Collection by endoscopy requires specialized equipment and it is not always easy to get liquid for culture; inaccurate results will be caused by dilution with gastric, biliary and pancreatic secretions, and accurate quantitative culture requires immediate access to an anaerobic chamber. This test is limited to academic institutions. The cut-offs for normal values are controversial. Total numbers of bacteria $>10^5$/ml, or $>10^4$/ml anaerobes, are considered diagnostic, but similar numbers may be found in asymptomatic dogs.
• Breath hydrogen. Measurement of breath hydrogen excretion is used as an indicator of SIBO, as hydrogen exhaled in the breath comes from intestinal bacterial fermentation. SIBO may be indicated by a raised resting breath hydrogen or by an early peak following oral administration of carbohydrate (e.g. xylose, lactulose). Similar results are seen if there is significant carbohydrate malabsorption or rapid small intestinal transit with increased colonic fermentation. The interpretation of results remains controversial.
• Folate and cobalamin. Small intestinal bacteria synthesize folate which is absorbed but bind cobalamin making it unavailable for absorption. Finding a raised serum folate and decreased cobalamin is suggestive of SIBO. Although quite specific, this result has a sensitivity of only 5%. The sensitivity of either just a raised folate or decreased cobalamin (51% and 24% respectively) is better but their specificities (79% and 87%) are much poorer. Thus SIBO cannot be diagnosed or ruled out based on folate and cobalamin alone.
• Antibiotic responsiveness. A consistent, positive response to antibiotics is suggestive but not diagnostic of SIBO; neither can it differentiate between idiopathic and secondary SIBO. In addition, a response to metronidazole may reflect its effect on *Giardia* or cell-mediated immunity rather than its antibacterial action.

117 A six-year-old, neutered male cat presented with an enlarged abdomen. On physical examination the abdomen could be balloted. There was the suggestion that the fluid was contained within defined areas; however, individual fluid-filled structures could not be palpated. The cat was depressed but otherwise unremarkable. Plain abdominal radiography

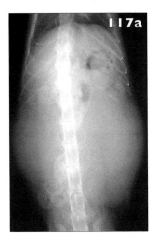 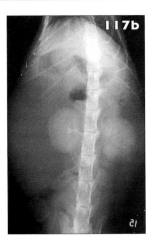

(117a) and intravenous urography (117b) were performed. Serum biochemical values were: urea 16 mmol/l, creatinine 200 mmol/l. Urine SG was 1.014. All other routine parameters were normal. Paracentesis of the mass on the right was performed and a clear fluid was obtained. The fluid had the appearance of a modified transudate (few mononuclear and polymorphonuclear cells, low in protein).
i. Describe the radiographs.
ii. What is your interpretation of the clinical pathology results?
iii. What is your diagnosis?

118 A ten-year-old, entire male Lhasa Apso was reported by the owner to be dribbling urine from the penis for one week. The owner was unsure if the dog had been urinating normally. A urethral catheter could not be passed when trying to obtain a urine sample. A plain radiograph was taken of the abdomen (118a).
i. What can you see on the film?
ii. How would you manage this dog?

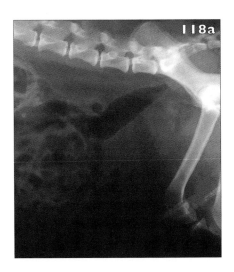

113

117 i. The plain radiograph shows two large, discrete, oval homogeneous soft tissue masses overlying the renal areas. These masses have well-defined smooth borders. Following intravenous administration of a contrast agent, small kidneys are visible within the soft tissue masses.

ii. The clinical pathology is consistent with mild primary renal failure. Although the urea and creatinine values are consistent with both primary renal failure and pre-renal azotaemia, the inappropriately dilute urine is indicative of a primary renal problem. Transudates result from increased capillary pressure, increased interstitial fluid pressure, a decrease in plasma oncotic pressure and an increase in interstitial oncotic pressure. In this case the fluid-filled structures are in a perirenal position and would therefore be consistent with a localized fluid production/resorption disorder. The fluid is not consistent with an infectious/inflammatory problem.

iii. An exploratory laparotomy revealed two fluid-filled sacs enclosing both kidneys. The diagnosis was perinephric pseudocysts. These are rare abnormalities. The fluid, which may be urine, blood, lymph or transudate, collects in the space between the renal capsule and the renal reflection of the peritoneum. Potential causes include trauma, surgery, neoplasia, venous congestion and hypertension. Affected cats are usually old and have concomitant renal disease. In this case no cause was determined. Renal function returned to normal once the fluid was removed.

118 i. The film shows multiple small radiodensities occluding the distal urethra caudal to the os penis, but the bladder is not particularly distended. This is compatible with partial urethral obstruction with calculi. Their radiographic density suggests the calculi are most likely to be struvite or oxalate. The stomach contains a large amount of ingesta.

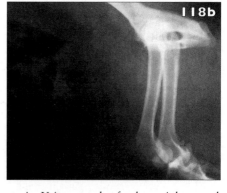

ii. The dog should be starved. The size of the bladder should be reassessed from a radiograph or by careful palpation and, if necessary, emptied by cystocentesis. Urine samples for bacteriology and urinalysis should be obtained, preferably by cystocentesis. As the dog is partially obstructed it is unlikely to be azotaemic and hyperkalaemic but routine haematology and biochemistry should be performed. With minimal delay, attempts should be made under general anaesthesia to return the calculi to the bladder by retrograde hydropropulsion (118b). Positive contrast urethrography and double contrast cystography should be considered to check for other lesions within the bladder and urethra which might have predisposed to calculi formation and obstruction. Once all the calculi are within the bladder a cystotomy should be performed, care being taken to remove all the calculi. The calculi should be submitted for qualitative analysis so that constructive advice can be given for the dog's future management.

Column A	Column B
i. Cholecystokinin ii. Motilin iii. Gastrin iv. Pepsin v. HCl vi. Secretin	a. Hormone synthesized and secreted in the gastric antrum to initiate release of gastric acid. b. Stimulates contraction of the gallbladder. c. Released in response to acidic chyme entering the intestine and stimulates pancreatic secretion of bicarbonate. d. Released from parietal cells in response to gastrin. e. The primary proteolytic enzyme in gastric juice. f. Initiates interdigestive intestinal motility, the effect of which is mimicked by low-dose erythromycin therapy (0.5–1.0 mg/kg p/o q8h).

119 Match the GI substance in column A to its appropriate description in column B.

120 A 13-year-old, neutered male foreign short-hair cat is presented for intermittent vomiting and weight loss of five months' duration. The vomitus usually contains malodorous food, and the timing of the vomiting bears no relationship to feeding. The owner also reports occasional bouts of diarrhoea, dullness and intermittent swelling of the abdomen. An abdominal radiograph was taken 17 hours after the administration of ten large and 30 small barium impregnated polyspheres (BIPS) (120).
i. What does the radiograph show?
ii. What are the possible causes/prognosis for this cat's signs?

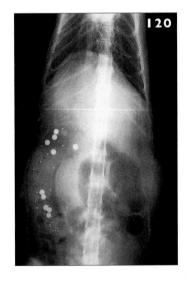

121 You obtain a blood sample from an eight-year-old, male crossbreed dog. The serum obtained from the sample was white due to lipaemia.
i. What is hyperlipaemia?
ii. Which two lipids are involved in normal body metabolism?
iii. Which lipid is responsible for lipaemia?
iv. What conditions might you associate with hyperlipaemia?

119 i. – b.
ii. – f.
iii. – a.
iv. – e.
v. – d.
vi. – c.

120 i. The BIPS are all collected in a grossly dilated loop of small intestine. This demonstrates severe, partial small intestinal obstruction.
ii. The major causes for small intestinal obstruction would be a foreign body, intussusception, inflammatory polyp or neoplasia. In view of the cat's age and the duration of clinical signs, intestinal neoplasia would be the most likely cause. At exploratory laparotomy an annular mass was found constricting the small intestine just distal to the dilated loop, which was accompanied by mesenteric lymphadenomegaly and multiple small white nodules throughout the mesentery over the parietal peritoneal surface. These findings are typical of small intestinal adenocarcinoma, which was confirmed by histological examination of the affected tissue.

Adenocarcinoma is the most common intestinal tumour in cats, and these tumours often grow relatively slowly resulting in a chronic history. By the time the disease is diagnosed, local and or distant metastases are common, as in this case, necessitating euthanasia. If an early diagnosis is made, and a solitary tumour identified, radical surgical resection may be curative. Chemotherapy or radiotherapy is considered to have little or no benefit.

121 i. Hyperlipaemia represents a disturbance of lipid transport due to either increased synthesis or decreased degradation of circulating lipoproteins.
ii. Triglycerides and cholesterol.
iii. Lipids are insoluble in plasma and thus they are transported in combination with protein as lipoproteins. Chylomicron and very low density lipoproteins contain mainly triglycerides. They are large and refract light and are thus responsible for the appearance of lipaemic plasma. Low density lipoproteins and high density lipoproteins transport predominantly cholesterol. They are small and do not refract light and thus hypercholesterolaemia never causes plasma to appear lipaemic.
iv. Idiopathic hyperlipidaemia; idiopathic hypercholesterolaemia; postprandial hyperlipidaemia; diabetes mellitus; hyperadrenocorticism; hypothyroidism; protein-losing nephropathy.

122 These kidneys are from a three-week-old Boxer puppy that died (122). All four of its littermates died as well. Prior to death they developed diarrhoea, which was yellow-green, showed distended abdomens and were crying.
i. What is your diagnosis?
ii. What spirochaete has been associated with renal failure in dogs?
iii. What is the treatment for this infection?
iv. What viral organisms may be associated with renal failure in cats?

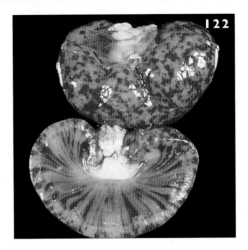

123 This nine-year-old, entire female Cavalier King Charles Spaniel (123) presented with a history of snoring, exercise intolerance and collapse. Collapsing episodes occurred at exercise and were characterized by flaccid muscles. The bitch recovered from the periods of collapse over one minute. She had previously been diagnosed as suffering from epilepsy and had been treated with phenobarbitone. This had resulted in marked depression. On presentation the bitch was overweight, tachycardic and had widening of the interdental spaces. Under a general anaesthetic an exuberance of oropharyngeal tissues and an overlong soft palate were present. Radiography demonstrated a mild cardiomegaly, hepatomegaly and renomegaly. Blood biochemistry is shown. Urine SG was 1.015 and urinalysis was otherwise unremarkable.
i. What condition(s) might you suspect?
ii. How might you pursue the diagnosis?
iii. What are the causes of this condition, and how might you treat them?

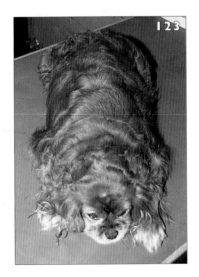

ALT (u/l)	120
ALP (u/l)	520
Bile acids (μmol/l)	4.9
Glucose (mmol/l)	10.2
Urea (mmol/l)	13
Creatinine (μmol/l)	200

122 i. Canine herpesvirus infection.

ii. *Leptospira.*

iii. The treatment for leptospiraemia may include use of procaine penicillin (20,000 u/kg i/m or s/c q12h for 14 days or until no azotaemia), tetracycline (5–10 mg/kg i/v q12h) or chloramphenicol (50 mg/kg i/v q8h). The treatment to eliminate the carrier state may include use of dihydrostreptomycin (10–15 mg/kg i/m q12h for 14 days) or doxycycline (5 mg/kg p/o as a loading dose, then 2.5 mg/kg q12h p/o for 2 weeks, then 2.5 mg/kg p/o q24h for 2 weeks).

iv. Feline infectious peritonitis, feline immunodeficiency virus.

123 i. The physical findings of an increase in organ size, overgrowth of soft tissues and increased bone growth (causing widening of the interdental spaces) is suggestive of acromegaly (excess growth hormone production). Biochemically there is a mild hyperglycaemia, mild renal failure (possibly pre-renal in origin) and evidence of a mild hepatopathy (hepatocellular damage and cholestasis), results which are also consistent with acromegaly.

ii. The diagnosis may be confirmed by assessing growth hormone (GH) production using a xylazine stimulation test. A ratio of GH post-stimulation:basal GH of >3.4 is consistent with acromegaly. In this bitch the ratio was 45.2. Demonstration of elevated plasma insulin growth factor may be used as an indicator of elevated plasma GH levels.

iii. Growth hormone overproduction has been associated with high progestagen concentrations, e.g. during dioestrus or as a result of treatment with progestagens such as medroxyprogesterone acetate. In some cases this results in insulin-resistant diabetes mellitus, with or without signs of acromegaly. Removal of the source of the progestagen, e.g. ovariohysterectomy, is indicated. Alternatively, it may develop as a consequence of a GH-producing pituitary tumour. This bitch failed to improve after ovariohysterectomy and thus a pituitary lesion was suspected, for which no treatment is currently available. CT/MRI scanning may be helpful in demonstrating a pituitary mass.

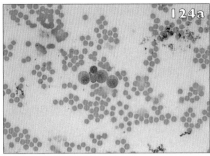

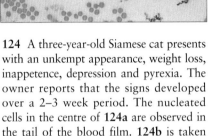

124 A three-year-old Siamese cat presents with an unkempt appearance, weight loss, inappetence, depression and pyrexia. The owner reports that the signs developed over a 2–3 week period. The nucleated cells in the centre of **124a** are observed in the tail of the blood film. **124b** is taken from the body of the film.
i. Identify the nucleated cells in **124a**.
ii. What is their significance?
iii. Comment on the RBC morphology in **124b**.
iv. What is the significance of this morphology?
   The haematological profile is shown.
v. What diagnostic test is indicated?

RBCs ($\times 10^9$/l)	3.05
Hb (g/l)	49
PCV (l/l)	0.21
MCV (fl)	67
MCHC (g/l)	240
nRBCs	7%
WBCs ($\times 10^9$/l)	12.8
Neutrophils (seg) ($\times 10^9$/l)	8.3
Neutrophils (bands) ($\times 10^9$/l)	0.24
Lymphocytes ($\times 10^9$/l)	1.4
Monocytes ($\times 10^9$/l)	1.71
Eosinophils ($\times 10^9$/l)	0.13
Others ($\times 10^9$/l)	0.13

Comment: blasts 1%; nRBCs at various stages; platelets appear low in the film.

125 A 16-week-old, male mixed breed terrier presented with a three-week history of vomiting and weight loss. He had a ravenous appetite but was unable to retain food and occasionally water without vomiting immediately after feeding. An abdominal radiograph is shown (**125a**).
i. What is your diagnosis?
ii. How will you approach this problem?

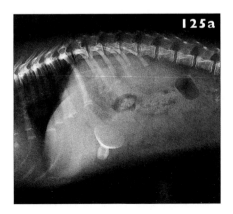

124 i. The four cells at the centre of the figure are erythroid precursors; there are three prorubricytes sandwiching a polychromatic rubricyte.

ii. The presence of nRBCs in the circulation is always abnormal. The presence of earlier erythroid precursors than metarubricytes (i.e. rubricytes, prorubricytes or rubriblasts) is usually due to bone marrow disease/damage, although these can sometimes be seen when there is marked extramedullary haematopoiesis, splenic dysfunction or splenectomy.

iii. Apart from the presence of nRBCs, the red cell morphology is normal, i.e. no anisocytosis or polychromasia.

iv. The lack of polychromasia and the presence of nRBCs confirms that this is not a regenerative response but is an abnormality of erythrocyte maturation and release into the peripheral circulation.

v. This macrocytic non-regenerative anaemia and thrombocytopenia, with occasional blast cells and large numbers of nRBCs at various stages of maturation in the circulation, is typical of FeLV-associated bone marrow disease. Assessment for FeLV antigen is indicated. It was positive in this case.

125 i. A suction cup-shaped foreign body is seen in the pyloric region of the stomach. On questioning, the owner stated that her son had been missing an 'arrow-head' from his toy set for several weeks.

ii. It is unlikely that a foreign body of this size will pass through the pylorus and/or intestine without causing further problems. Options for removal include retrieval via endoscopy or by surgical gastrostomy. The less invasive method of endoscopy was chosen with a view to pursuing surgery if the object proved too large or was not amenable to endoscopic removal. The endoscopic appearance of the object completely obstructing the pylorus is shown (**125b**). The object was circled with basket retrieval forceps and easily retracted through the oral cavity.

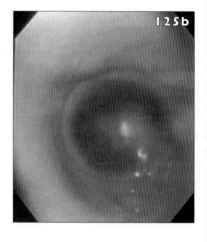

126 A six-month-old, male Great Dane presented with a history of recurrent urinary tract infections despite several courses of antibiotics. The urine persistently had a foul smell and the owner had noticed fluid with the appearance of urine leaking from the dog's anus after micturition. Clinical examination was unremarkable.

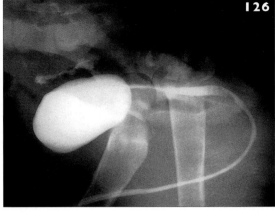

i. List the diagnostic investigations you would perform on this dog.

This radiograph (**126**) was obtained.

ii. What is your diagnosis?

iii. How would you treat the dog?

127 A two-year-old, male German Shepherd Dog had chronic diarrhoea and profound weight loss (from 45 kg to 36 kg in six weeks) despite a ravenous appetite (**127a**). Excessive borborygmi and flatus were noted and the dog was coprophagic. Serum folate was increased (13.5 µg/l) and cobalamin decreased (35 ng/l), and a presumptive diagnosis of small intestinal bacterial overgrowth (SIBO) was made. Treatment with oxytetracycline resulted in better stool consistency but

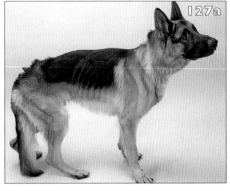

no weight gain. Routine haematology had initially shown an absolute eosinophil count of 1.5×10^9/l and, on the assumption that this was an indicator of eosinophilic enteritis, the dog was then started on immunosuppressive doses of prednisolone. The diarrhoea worsened and despite increasing the dosage of prednisolone the weight fell rapidly to 23 kg.

Why did treatment fail in this dog, and what test would have given the correct diagnosis?

126 i. • Haematology and biochemistry.
• Urine bacteriology and urinalysis.
• Observe urination and possibly collect fluid passed from anus for analysis.
• Positive contrast retrograde urethrocystogram and double contrast cystogram.
• Ultrasound examination of the kidneys, bladder and prostate. This allows determination of changes affecting the upper urinary tract and prostate which may be the result of chronic urinary tract infection.
ii. The history is suggestive of a congenital urethrorectal fistula and associated urinary tract infection. The presence and the position of a urethrorectal fistula is confirmed in the radiograph (**126**).
iii. Surgical closure of the fistula. In this dog the fistula was positioned within the pelvic canal and a sagittal pubic osteotomy was used to reach the fistula. Congenital fistulas are usually well-defined tubes; in this case the fistula was isolated and ligated at each end before being sectioned. Once the fistula has been closed the urinary tract infection should be treated using an antibiotic based on culture and sensitivity. It is important that an adequate dose of the drug is given for long enough to eradicate the infection. Following antibiotic treatment, repeat urine cultures should be performed to ensure that the infection has been eradicated. In this case the dog was treated with a three-week course of enrofloxacin; urine culture one week after the course finished produced no bacterial growth. Following surgery the dog was continent.

127 The clinical signs of chronic diarrhoea, weight loss, ravenous appetite and coprophagia are consistent with SIBO or exocrine pancreatic insufficiency (EPI). A trypsin-like immunoreactivity (TLI) test should have been performed before primary intestinal disease was assumed. Although SIBO is a frequent complication of EPI, serum folate and cobalamin abnormalities are commonly seen in EPI and are not necessarily indicative of SIBO, as normal

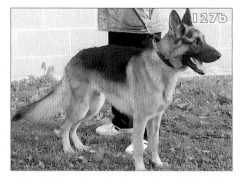

pancreatic secretions are involved in the absorption of cobalamin in particular. The TLI in this dog (0.3 µg/l) was diagnostic for EPI, and the borborygmi, flatus, watery diarrhoea and partial response to antibiotics were suggestive of secondary SIBO. This would be expected to worsen when steroids are administered.

While inflammatory changes in the intestinal mucosa can be seen in EPI, eosinophilia is a very unreliable marker of eosinophilic enteritis, and in the German Shepherd Dog this degree of eosinophilia is considered by some to be normal for the breed. This case highlights the dangers of giving corticosteroids without biopsy proof of inflammatory bowel disease. The dog was weaned off all steroids and given pancreatic enzyme replacement and oxytetracycline. Within six weeks it had gained 9 kg and ultimately returned to 42 kg body weight (**127b**).

128 A two-year-old dog presents with a four-week history of vomiting undigested food and water minutes to hours after eating, and hypersalivation. He is thin, keen to eat and has halitosis. Diarrhoea and exercise intolerance are not reported. Serum biochemistry and haematology are unremarkable. Barium sulphate is administered and this radiograph obtained (**128**).

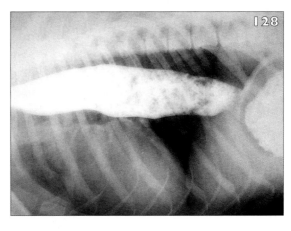

i. What abnormalities do you recognize?
ii. What diagnosis would you make?
iii. What other diagnostic tests might you consider?
iv. How would you manage this case?

129 An 11-year-old, female neutered Golden Retriever presented with acute urinary tract obstruction. Clinical examination was unremarkable apart from the presence of a full bladder and a pea-sized urethral mass palpated on rectal and vaginal examination.
i. What are your differential diagnoses?

After emptying the bladder, plain abdominal and

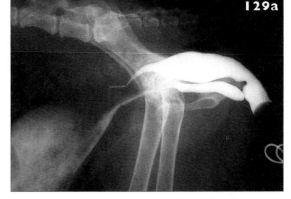

positive contrast vagino-urethrogram (**129a**) radiographic examinations were performed.
ii. How would you further investigate this dog?

128 i. The radiograph shows a dilated oesophagus. The dilation extends throughout the length of the oesophagus.
ii. Megaoesophagus.
iii. The cause of the generalized megaoesophagus was not determined. Endoscopic examination of the oesophagus, stomach and duodenum only served to confirm the presence of the megaoesophagus; no obstructive lesions were seen. Fluoroscopically, the oesophagus was noted to be very hypomotile.
iv. The prognosis is poor. Management is aimed at feeding from an elevated or upright position to aid passage of food into the stomach. A solid (not liquidized) food high in energy is fed so as to maximize energy intake.

129 i. The main differential diagnoses are: urethral neoplasia; urethral calculus; granulomatous urethritis; bladder neoplasia; vaginal neoplasia obstructing the external urethral orifice or compressing the urethra intrapelvically.
ii. Investigations which should be performed on this dog are:
• Obtain urine samples by cystocentesis for bacteriology and urinalysis prior to catheterization.

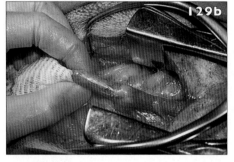

• Routine haematology and biochemistry to check the animals general health and presence of azotaemia and hyperkalaemia.
• The contrast radiograph shows the urethral contrast column abruptly narrowing within the pelvis at a site which corresponded with the palpable mass. Further radiographic investigations would include a double contrast cystogram and thoracic films to check for metastatic spread in cases of suspected neoplasia.
• Ultrasound examination of the caudal abdomen is a useful technique for examining the bladder for the presence of masses as well as checking the sublumbar lymph nodes for enlargement and the liver for focal lesions suggestive of metastases, although in this case no abnormalities were seen. It may be used to obtain guided catheter biopsies from some bladder lesions.
• Biopsy of any masses/irregularities in the urethral lumen. In the absence of a cystoscope allowing direct biopsy, lesions within the urethra are most easily sampled using a catheter biopsy technique. In some cases, such as this (**129b**), an excisional biopsy was possible.

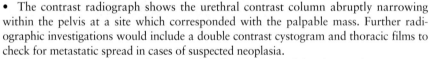

	Cat 1	Cat 2	Cat 3
ALP (u/l)	350	28	510
ALT (u/l)	236	164	461
GGT (u/l)	2	1	13

130 Match the serum liver enzyme activities with the description of the animal they most likely represent, and give a short explanation of the pathogenesis for these changes or the lack thereof. For each cat there is a corresponding best matching set of values.

a. Eight-year-old, female Persian with a distended abdomen, hyperglobulinaemia and hepatomegaly. Abdominocentesis yields a viscous, proteinaceous exudate. Coronavirus titre is 1:3200.

b. Three-year-old, male, previously obese domestic longhair cat which is anorexic, has lost 1.5 kg body weight in three weeks and is clinically jaundiced. Hepatic biopsy reveals severe vacuolation of hepatocytes.

c. Fifteen-year-old, male domestic shorthair cat with weight loss, unkempt dry hair coat, polyphagia, tachycardia and a palpable thyroid nodule.

131 This 18-month-old, female Miniature Pinscher was referred with a six-month history of chronic intermittent diarrhoea with occasional fresh blood (**131a**). There had been no weight loss. Signs had started shortly after elective ovariohysterectomy. As they had improved every time antibiotics had been given, the referring veterinary surgeon had made a tentative diagnosis of idiopathic small intestinal bacterial overgrowth (SIBO). On physical examination the dog was slightly depressed and intermittently performed stretching motions as if there was some abdominal discomfort. Physical examination and vital

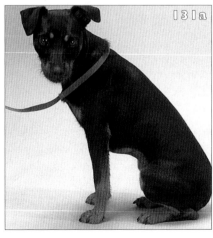

signs were normal, and routine haematology, serum biochemistry and serum folate and cobalamin were unremarkable.

i. Why is a diagnosis of idiopathic SIBO not justified in this case?
ii. How would you attempt to reach a definitive diagnosis?

130 Cat 1 – b. This history is typical of a cat with hepatic lipidosis and this would be supported by the finding of vacuolated hepatocytes and seemingly disparate results of serum liver enzyme activity. Although choices a. and c. would also be possible, an increased serum ALP concentration in conjunction with a normal serum GGT concentration is a common laboratory finding in cats with hepatic lipidosis.

Cat 2 – c. This cat has signs of feline hyperthyroidism which should be investigated with a basal serum thyroxine concentration. Hyperthyroidism commonly results in mild elevations of serum liver enzyme activities, specifically ALT. This biochemical abnormality usually resolves upon successful treatment.

Cat 3 – a. This cat may be infected with FIP and a liver biopsy would be necessary to confirm this suspicion. The increase in all three liver enzyme activities reflects an active disease process affecting the liver, which can occur with FIP infections.

131 i. The repeated response to antibiotics by this dog is consistent with SIBO (or perhaps infection with a specific pathogen such as *Campylobacter*), but SIBO is only definitively diagnosed by quantitative culture of duodenal juice. Furthermore, idiopathic SIBO is a diagnosis usually made in young, large breed dogs, especially German Shepherd Dogs, after underlying disease has been ruled out. In SIBO, signs of chronic intermittent diarrhoea may occur with or without weight loss, and whilst passage of fresh blood is not common, it can occur if bacterial metabolites cause a secondary colitis. The normal folate and cobalamin in this case do not rule out SIBO as the classical changes of increased folate and decreased cobalamin are only seen in the minority of cases. The stretching signs are indicative of intra-abdominal inflammation and/or adhesions and would not be expected in idiopathic SIBO. Any overgrowth in this case is likely to be secondary to an underlying cause, e.g. mucosal disease, partial intestinal obstruction or exocrine pancreatic insufficiency (EPI).

ii. The lack of weight loss would make EPI very unlikely; serum TLI was normal. Plain radiographs were not helpful, but contrast studies and ultrasound examination might have been useful. Upper and lower GI endoscopy was performed. The stomach and duodenum were normal, but a haemorrhagic mass was observed in the proximal colon and the normal ileocolic valve was not found. A chronic ileocolic intussusception was identified at laparotomy and resected (**131b**). The previous antibiotic-responsive diarrhoea is presumed to have been due to both localized disease and SIBO proximal to the partial obstruction.

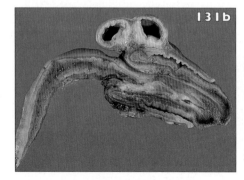

132 The haematological profile shown was obtained from an overweight, aged male Dobermann with a grade 3/6 murmur over the left heart base, petechiation and ecchymoses on the gums, conjunctiva and ear pinnae, mild pyrexia, left hind-limb lameness, testicular asymmetry, lethargy, pallor and reduced appetite.
i. How would you interpret this profile?
ii. What would be your next diagnostic step?

RBCs ($\times 10^{12}$/l)	2.71
Hb (g/l)	66
PCV (l/l)	0.22
MCV (fl)	82
MCHC (g/l)	300
nRBCs	6%
Platelets ($\times 10^9$/l)	1
WBCs ($\times 10^9$/l)	3.2
Neutrophils (seg) ($\times 10^9$/l)	2.2
Neutrophils (bands) ($\times 10^9$/l)	0.16
Lymphocytes ($\times 10^9$/l)	0.64
Monocytes ($\times 10^9$/l)	0.2

Comment: platelets very low in the film; polychromasia +/-; anisocytosis +/-.

133 An eight-year-old, male West Highland White Terrier presented with a three-week history of dysuria and haematuria. Ultrasound examination of the bladder revealed this lesion (**133**).
i. What can you see, and what is your differential diagnosis?
ii. How would you confirm your diagnosis?

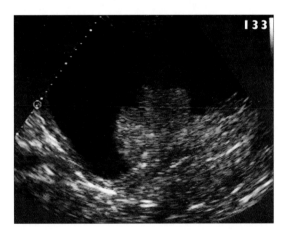

134 A nine-year-old domestic shorthair cat presents with a history of depression, weight loss (2.3 kg compared to its normal body weight of 4.4 kg) and inappetence of three weeks' duration. Vomiting and diarrhoea are not present. Rectal temperature is unremarkable. An abdominal mass is present and an exploratory laparotomy was scheduled to investigate the case further.
i. Are you concerned with this cat's nutritional status? If yes, why; if no, why not?
ii. How would you manage the cat nutritionally pre- and postoperatively?

132 i. This is a pancytopenia, i.e. neutropenia, lymphopenia, thrombocytopenia and poorly regenerative anaemia, indicative of bone marrow disease. The thrombocytopenia is very severe and explains the presence of petechiae and ecchymoses. There is a risk of spontaneous GI or CNS haemorrhage. The presence of nRBCs probably reflects bone marrow dysfunction rather than a coordinated regenerative response, as there are disproportionately large numbers of nRBCs compared to the amount of polychromasia.

ii. A bone marrow biopsy is indicated but the thrombocytopenia does constitute a significant risk for this procedure. Biopsy might be considered after a fresh blood or platelet-rich plasma transfusion. There is a much less invasive way of achieving a diagnosis in this case. The key is the presence of testicular asymmetry. The serum oestradiol concentration was markedly elevated at 320 pmol/l. From this it can be assumed that testicular asymmetry is due to the presence of a testicular tumour, probably a Sertoli cell tumour. The haematological findings are typical of long-standing oestrogen toxicosis.

133 i. A hyperechoic mass can be seen arising from the bladder wall and projecting into the bladder lumen. The margin of the mass is irregular and it involves and disrupts the normal layers of the bladder wall. The most likely differential diagnosis is a bladder wall neoplasm, e.g. transitional cell carcinoma, or a rhabdomyosarcoma. In this case a transitional cell carcinoma was considered most likely due to the involvement of the trigone, the dog's age and the irregular marginated appearance of the mass.

ii. The diagnosis should be confirmed histopathologically. Bladder masses may be biopsied using a catheter suction technique under ultrasound guidance. In this case a catheter was placed in the bladder and, by applying pressure to the caudal abdominal wall, the bladder wall could be pushed against the catheter. When the mass was in contact with the catheter, negative pressure was applied with a syringe and small amounts of tissue obtained by suction. Blind catheter suction is unreliable but in this case would probably have been possible due to the large size of the tumour. Cytological examination of urine sediment may reveal neoplastic transitional cells which have exfoliated from the mass. Tissue may also be obtained directly during surgery or, in female dogs, by cystoscopy. In this case the diagnosis of transitional carcinoma was confirmed.

134 i. This cat's main problem aside from the mass is severe protein-energy malnutrition (PEM). Traumatized patients, which includes those undergoing surgery, have increased requirements for energy and protein as a consequence of an increase in the metabolic rate that accompanies inflammation/stress. Mobilization of body tissue results, although feeding prior to the traumatic event and ensuring adequate nutrition postoperatively will ameliorate the effects of the PEM. If untreated, PEM may result in poor wound healing, organ failure, immunoincompetence and sepsis.

ii. This cat's plane of nutrition needs to be improved prior to surgery. It is not necessary to attain its optimal weight, only to ensure that the cat is on a rising plane of nutrition and is receiving adequate nutrition. An energy dense diet containing easily digestible high-quality nutrients should be fed until the metabolic consequences of the trauma have resolved. A nasogastric tube was placed one week pre-operatively and a high-energy, high-protein tubable diet administered. At laparotomy a gastrostomy tube was placed and the cat fed through this until it was able to consume sufficient food voluntarily.

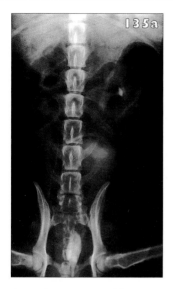

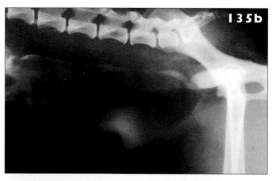

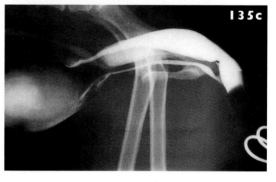

135 A two-year-old, entire female Border Terrier presented with chronic low-grade, dribbling incontinence since a pup. The dribbling varies little from day to day. The bitch urinates normally from the vulva, there have been no episodes of urinary tract infection and the bitch has had two normal seasons. The dog has received no medical treatment for the incontinence.

i. What are your three main differential diagnoses?

  Radiographic investigations were performed and an intravenous urogram and retrograde vagino-urethrogram obtained (135a–135c).

ii. What is your diagnosis?

iii. What treatment would you advise?

136 You have diagnosed gastric ulceration in a 12-year-old, neutered male, 28 kg Irish Setter. The dog had a history of acute vomiting 24 hours prior to being presented in a collapsed state. A transfusion of fresh whole blood was administered prior to endoscopic examination of the stomach. An ulcerated lesion was seen. A biopsy was reported as inflammation or reactive hyperplasia rather than neoplasia. The dog was receiving phenylbutazone for a chronic osteoarthritic disorder.

i. What treatment will you prescribe for this dog?

ii. What further follow-up would you recommend?

135 i. Ectopic ureter; urethral sphincter mechanism incompetence; congenital anatomical urogenital tract abnormality.

ii. A left ectopic ureter. The left ureter is moderately dilated along its length and terminates as a very small opening in the caudal vagina, dorsal to the external urethral orifice. There is a large ureterocele immediately dorsal to the bladder neck/proximal urethra. The bladder contains contrast medium and there is no evidence of a second ectopic ureter on the retrograde vagino-urethrogram. The right ureter was confirmed to enter the bladder normally on ultrasound examination. The bladder neck is intra-abdominal.

iii. Surgical reimplantation of the ureter into the bladder. In view of the ureterocele the tunnelling technique was considered the most appropriate method of reimplantation. As the dog only has one ectopic ureter and no evidence clinically or radiographically of urethral sphincter mechanism incompetence, a good prognosis for complete continence was given. This dog did not have a urinary tract infection. In the event of a urinary tract infection, treatment with an appropriate antibiotic is strongly advised before surgical treatment is performed.

136 i. Treatment of gastric ulceration requires identification and removal, if possible, of the underlying disorder. In this dog the use of phenylbutazone was discontinued. Fluids, including whole blood as needed, should be given to maintain fluid balance and restore gastric mucosal blood flow. Antibiotics may be indicated as mucosal disruption may serve as a site for bacterial translocation and sepsis. Secondary therapy includes decreasing gastric acidity and restoring normal gastric protective mechanisms such as replenishing the gastric mucous barrier and blood flow. H2-receptor antagonists e.g. cimetidine (5–10 mg/kg q8h), ranitidine (2 mg/kg q12h) or famotidine (0.5–1.0 mg/kg q24h), reduce acid production by blocking the histamine receptor of the parietal cell. Omeprazole (1–2 mg/kg p/o q24h) inhibits the proton pump and is a potent deterrent to gastric acid production. Oral antacids are unnecessary since the above medications are more effective in increasing gastric pH. Cytoprotective agents such as sucralfate (1 gm/30 kg p/o q8h) bind to denuded proteins at the site of ulceration and form a protective barrier. Prostaglandins and their synthetic analogues such as misoprostol (3–5 µg/kg p/o q8h) speed the rate of gastric healing, reduce gastric acid secretion and help prevent further ulcerations.

ii. To ensure that the lesion is healing appropriately prior to discontinuing the gastric protectant medications, the dog's stool should be closely observed for the presence of melena. Clinical signs such as vomiting and inappetence should resolve. A second endoscopic examination is performed to ensure that the ulcer is healing and that an underlying neoplastic disease has not been missed. Endoscopic examination four weeks later revealed a reduced, much less inflamed area of resolving hyperplastic tissue (**136**).

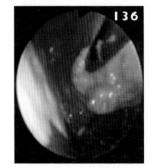

137 A 16-year-old, neutered male domestic shorthair cat presents with a four-day history of anorexia. Body weight is 3 kg. The cat is depressed and approximately 7% dehydrated. The kidneys are small. Vaccinations are up to date. Serum biochemistry, haematology and urinalysis are performed on day 1. Urine cytology is unremarkable.

i. What is your assessment of these results on day 1?

ii. Describe your fluid treatment plan?

Following fluid therapy urine output was estimated to be 11 ml/hr. Fluid rate was therefore increased to 11 ml/hr and urine output monitored overnight. The cat's body-weight increased from 3 kg to 3.2 kg (an increase of approximately 7%). On day 2 the cat was brighter and voluntarily drank water. Serum biochemistry was repeated on day 2 and abdominal radiography and ultrasonography were performed (137a–137c).

iii. What is your assessment?

iv. What is your treatment plan?

Over the next 24 hours, intravenous fluid therapy was gradually decreased and then discontinued. The cat was eating and drinking well and maintained a body weight of 3.2 kg. His laboratory evaluation at discharge (day 5) is shown.

v. What is your assessment?

vi. What is your follow-up plan?

	Day 1	Day 2	Day 5
Albumin (g/l)	39	29	
ALP (u/l)	16	6	
ALT (u/l)	67	46	
Total protein (g/l)	84	59	
Urea (mmol/l)	45	26	27
Creatinine (μmol/l)	663	336	327
Glucose (mmol/l)	6.8	7.3	7.0
Sodium (mmol/l)	162	151	150
Potassium (mmol/l)	5.0	4.1	4.5
Chloride (mmol/l)	131	125	120
Calcium (mmol/l)	2.8	2.4	2.5
Phosphorus (mmol/l)	3.2	1.6	1.5
Total CO_2 (mEq/l)	6.0	14	16
Anion gap (mEq/l)	31	16	18
PCV (l/l)	0.32		
WBCs ($\times 10^9$/l)	9.0		
White cell differential: unremarkable			

Urinalysis:

Colour/turbidity	Yellow/clear
SG	1.011
pH	6.0
Glucose, ketones, bilirubin	Negative
Occult blood	Negative
Protein – qualitative	Negative

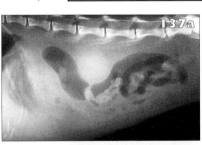

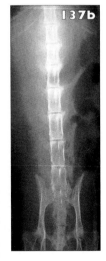

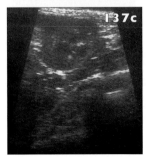

137 i. The presence of isosthenuria with azotaemia is most consistent with renal failure. Because the kidneys are palpably small and the PCV is low normal in the presence of dehydration, chronic renal failure with an acute decompensation is most likely.

ii. When formulating fluid treatment plans you must decide on the type of fluid (balanced electrolyte solution for rehydration, e.g. lactated Ringer's solution); the route of fluid administration (intravenous); and the rate of administration. The rate and amount of fluid is determined by three factors:

- Rehydration: volume required = % body weight loss × body weight (kg) = 7% × 3 kg = 210 ml. Rehydrate over 8 hours, therefore 26.25 ml/hr.
- Maintenance requirements = 2.2 ml/kg/hr = 2.2 × 3 = 6.6 ml/hr.
- Ongoing losses = amount lost via vomiting, diarrhoea, etc. = 0 ml/hr.

Therefore, administer approximately 33 ml/hr of lactated Ringer's solution i/v for eight hours, then reduce to maintenance (7 ml/hr). After a couple of hours of maintenance fluid therapy, assess urine production by observing urination in a litter pan, palpating the bladder or weighing absorbent pads used to line the floor of the cage (weight of urine soaked pad minus weight of pad [approximately 20 g] = g[ml] of urine voided).

iii. Because the cat is still azotaemic following rehydration and fluid therapy, in addition to the small appearance of the kidneys on radiographs and ultrasound, the renal failure is likely to be chronic in nature.

iv. Fluid therapy could be slowly discontinued with continued monitoring of the azotaemia.

v. The degree of azotaemia is probably stable and approximately what it was prior to the episode of acute renal failure. Therefore, the cat probably had an episode of acute renal failure in addition to his chronic renal failure.

vi. Follow-up plans should include periodic monitoring of clinical findings and laboratory work to evaluate the development of dehydration, malnutrition, electrolyte imbalances (hypokalaemia), metabolic acidosis and neuroendocrine imbalances (hypoproliferative anaemia, hyperphosphataemia, systemic hypertension) which may alter the course of the renal failure. Furthermore, efforts should be made to minimize exposure to other renal insults such as nephrotoxins and hypoperfusion.

138 These bladder stones (**138**) were removed via cystotomy from a 16-month-old, female Yorkshire Terrier with chronic intermittent dysuria and haematuria. Abdominal radiographs had not shown evidence for calculi but uroliths were discovered during ovariohysterectomy. The dog was small for its age and took a long time to recover from

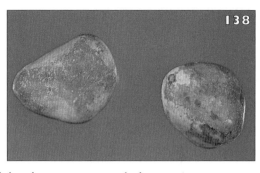

anaesthesia. Stone analysis revealed that they were composed of ammonium urate.
i. What is the significance of urate urolithiasis in this dog?
ii. What tests would you do to confirm your diagnosis?
iii. How can you prevent recurrence of urate urolithiasis in this patient?

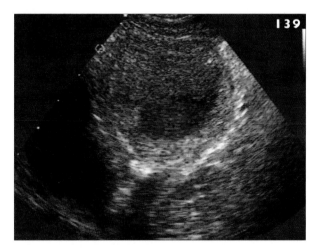

139 A 12-year-old, entire male Labrador presented with a two-day history of dysuria following a recent bout of vomiting and diarrhoea. The owner reported that the dog was lethargic and anorexic. Clinical examination revealed the dog to be pyrexic with a rectal temperature of 40.3°C (104.5°F).
i. What are your three most likely differential diagnoses?
ii. How would you investigate this dog further?
iii. What features do you recognize in the ultrasound image of the prostate (**139**)?

138 i. Urate uroliths are found rarely in non-Dalmatian dogs, except in dogs with congenital portosystemic shunts. In these dogs, reduced liver function leads to decreased hepatic conversion of uric acid to allantoin and ammonia to urea. Urolithiasis is sometimes the main or only presenting sign. Urate stones tend to be radiolucent and are only seen on contrast radiography or ultrasonography. The history of stunted growth and slow anaesthetic recovery (suggestive of impaired hepatic metabolism) might also point towards a possible congenital portosystemic shunt.

ii. The next step should be to look for underlying liver disease and/or portosystemic shunting. It is advisable to wait at least two weeks after surgery before blood testing in order to reduce interference by anaesthesia and surgery. Fasting and postprandial serum bile acids should be determined and, if possible, blood ammonia concentration. Urinalysis and culture should be undertaken to rule out urinary tract infection, which may exacerbate urolithiasis. Hepatic ultrasonography can identify a portosystemic shunt but requires an experienced ultrasonographer.

iii. Surgical ligation of a congenital portosystemic shunt will help to prevent recurrence of urate lithiasis. Existing stones usually have to be removed surgically.

139 i. Prostatic abscess; acute prostatitis; urinary tract infection.

ii. • Prostatic palpation to assess for enlargement, asymmetry, pain and fluctuant swelling. In this case the prostate was intra-abdominal and not palpable per rectum. An apple-sized mass could be palpated in the caudal abdomen.

• Routine haematology and biochemistry.

• Urinalysis and bacteriology.

• Plain radiograph of the abdomen to check prostate size, and look for evidence of localized or generalized peritonitis and other abdominal disease.

• Ultrasound examination of the prostate provides useful information on the size and texture of the prostate as well as revealing cysts or abscess cavities. It allows ultrasound-guided aspiration of any cystic lesions seen.

• Contrast studies of the lower urinary tract (retrograde urethrocystogram and double contrast cystogram) allow full examination of the urethra and should reveal communications between prostatic cystic lesions and the urethra. This information is important when considering the most appropriate surgical management.

• If treated surgically, biopsies should always be taken from the wall of prostatic cysts and abscesses as occasionally they occur in conjunction with neoplasia.

iii. A cystic lesion is arising from the prostate. Aspiration of the lesion produced pus and a diagnosis of prostatic abscess was confirmed. Ultrasound-guided aspiration of prostatic abscesses is an area of controversy with some clinicians advising against the procedure in case pus leakage results in peritonitis. However, the author has found no such complications. Samples obtained should be submitted for bacteriology and cytology.

	Calcium (mmol/l)	Phosphate (mmol/l)	Parathyroid hormone (PTH) (pmol/l)
A	4.2	0.6	30
B	2.7	4.8	24
C	4.1	0.43	2.3
D	3.2	1.3	3.5
E	1.7	2.1	25
F	4.9	3.8	<1

140 Match each of the six sets of results above with the appropriate diagnosis/clinical description. Some result sets may apply to more than one diagnosis, therefore choose what you see as the best fit.

i. A seven-year-old dog with chronic PU/PD of several months' duration, anorexia, weight loss, drowsiness, urine SG 1.014, blood urea 34 mmol/l, creatinine 400 µmol/l and ananaemia (PCV 0.22l/l).

ii. A four-year-old male dog with a small pea-like mass in the region of the anal glands and a sublumbar lymphadenopathy on abdominal radiography.

iii. A thirteen-year-old dog with PU/PD of a few weeks' duration, inappetence, weight loss, urine SG 1.011, blood urea 20 mmol/l, creatinine 200 µmol/l.

iv. An adult dog with acute onset depression, weakness and anorexia. Exposure to cholecalciferol rodenticides was a possibility. Biochemistry results were urea 60 mmol/l, creatinine 900 mmol/l. Urine SG was 1.025.

v. A three-year-old Retriever with a chronic history of intermittent vomiting and diarrhoea and occasional weakness and exercise intolerance. On physical examination a mild bradycardia is present. Urea 18 mmol/l, creatinine 200 µmol/l, potassium 5.9 mmol/l, sodium 138 mmol/l.

vi. A six-month-old crossbreed dog with acute right hindlimb lameness. Radiography shows the bone cortices to be thin and a pathological fracture in the right tibia. The dog was fed exclusively an all-meat diet.

141 A six-month-old, male German Shepherd Dog with chronic diarrhoea has grossly (**141**) and microscopically normal intestine on endoscopic biopsy. Small intestinal bacterial overgrowth (SIBO) is confirmed by quantitative culture of duodenal juice (1.2×10^8 cfu/ml).

How would you treat idiopathic SIBO?

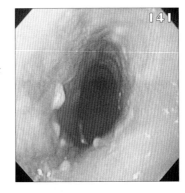

140 i. B. The history is typical of chronic renal failure. In such cases serum calcium may be low, normal or high, but phosphate is usually elevated. With the development of renal secondary hyperparathyroidism, PTH is also increased.

ii. C. Apocrine carcinomas of the anal glands often produce a PTH-related protein which acts like PTH to promote hypercalcaemia and hypophosphataemia. Unlike primary hyperparathyroidism, the PTH concentrations are low. These tumours often metastasize to sublumbar lymph nodes.

iii. A. Primary hyperparathyroidism can present with various signs ranging from vague signs of inappetence and mild PU/PD to severe renal failure or coma. Distinguishing primary hypoparathyroidism from chronic renal failure can be difficult. However, as a general but not exclusive rule, serum phosphate values are low with primary hypoparathyroidism but high with chronic renal failure. The other clinical pathological features can be identical, although hypercalcaemia is an unusual finding in chronic renal failure.

iv. F. Cholecalciferol rodenticides cause severe hypercalcaemia and hyperphosphataemia which can result in acute renal failure. The main differential diagnoses are hypoadrenocorticism and chronic renal failure (CRF). However, the low PTH would rule out CRF and the hypercalcaemia associated with hypoadrenocorticism is usually only mild.

v. D. The vague clinical signs and the serum biochemistry would be consistent with hypoadrenocorticism. Mild hypercalcaemia and hyperphosphataemia may be recognized. Serum PTH would be expected to be normal or slightly low.

vi. E. The history is typical of secondary nutritional hyperparathyroidism. In such cases the PTH is driven high by the imbalanced calcium:phosphorus ratio associated with consumption of a meat only diet. Calcium and phosphate may be normal or low.

141 Provided there is no underlying cause, treatment is based on long-term, broad-spectrum antibiotic administration. Oxytetracycline (10–20 mg/kg p/o q8h) is preferred, based on relative cost and likelihood of success, but other antibiotics such as metronidazole (10–20 mg/kg p/o q8h), amoxycillin (10 mg/kg p/o q8h) or tylosin (10 mg/kg p/o q8h) can be tried. At least four weeks medication is given assuming a positive initial response. Immediate relapse on cessation of antibiotics may occur in some cases and, assuming no treatable underlying cause can be found, continuous antibiotics may be required for control. Empirically, it may be possible to reduce antibiotic dosage frequency to twice daily or even once daily and maintain control. A highly digestible low-fat diet is a useful adjunct to antibiotic therapy, and indeed may be the only treatment needed in mild cases. Addition of novel carbohydrates (fructo-oligosaccharides) to the diet to control the bacterial flora has not yet been proven to be effective. Similarly, probiotics are unlikely to be helpful. In many cases, serum cobalamin is markedly reduced and parenteral administration of cobalamin (250–500 μg s/c monthly) may be beneficial.

142 A nine-year-old, male crossbreed presented with depression, lethargy and loss of appetite of two days' duration. The dog had been drinking excessively for some months, although this had not worried the owner, and he had a good appetite until recently. Bilateral cataracts (142) had developed over the preceding two months. The retina could not be visualized. There was no evidence of glaucoma or of any problem with the anterior chamber. On abdominal palpation the liver was palpably enlarged and the dog was 5% dehydrated. Clinical biochemistry values are shown.

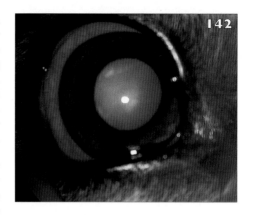

i. What is your interpretation of the clinical biochemistry, and what are your main differential diagnoses?
ii. Are further tests in order, or would you treat the patient?

Sodium (mmol/l)	145
Potassium (mmol/l)	5.9
Calcium (mmol/l)	2.2
Glucose (mmol/l)	28.9
Beta-hydroxybutyrate (mmol/l)	2.1
Urea (mmol/l)	11
Creatinine (µmol/l)	100
Phosphate (mmol/l)	1.5
ALT (u/l)	60
ALP (u/l)	800
SIAP (%)	65
Bile acids (µmol/l)	12
Cholesterol (mmol/l)	10.1
Total protein (g/l)	65
Albumin (g/l)	30

143 A dog is diagnosed as having a ureterolith with ureteral obstruction and mild hydronephrosis. Urinalysis revealed: pH 6.5; SG 1.045; dipstick negative for bilirubin, glucose and ketones; protein 2+; and occult blood 2+. Cytological examination of the sediment of a centrifuged urine sample revealed 50–100 RBCs/hpf, 1–5 WBCs/hpf and no bacteria or crystals.
i. What is the likely composition of the urolith?
ii. How does this urolith form?
iii. What is the long-term preventive treatment?

142 i. There are marked increases in blood glucose, ketones, ALP and SIAP. The elevated blood glucose is consistent with diabetes mellitus. Ketosis develops as a consequence of cellular starvation and in small animals is most commonly seen in insulin deficient animals. The elevated ALP is indicative of a mild hepatopathy (cholestasis, hepatocellular damage). However, the normal ALT would suggest that there is no ongoing hepatocellular damage and there is no evidence of hepatic dysfunction (normal bile acids). Cholestasis may be seen in animals with diabetes mellitus due to hepatic lipid deposition. The increase in SIAP is consistent with induction of ALP production by corticosteroids. Although this may raise the suspicion of hyperadrenocorticism (HAC), it is not a specific feature for this disease, with other causes of hepatic disease (including diabetes mellitus) also resulting in elevated blood levels of this isoenzyme. Hypercholesterolaemia is a feature of deranged fat metabolism and is associated with several conditions including diabetes mellitus, HAC and hypothyroidism. Hyperkalaemia is a feature of diabetes mellitus, particularly if ketoacidosis is present. The history, physical findings and clinical pathology are most consistent with diabetes mellitus, although HAC should also be considered.
ii. The findings so far are sufficient to make the diagnosis of diabetes mellitus. As artefactual results may be seen and given that treatment for diabetes mellitus may cause hypoglycaemia, documentation of a persistent hyperglycaemia is indicated in most cases. In this case, prompt treatment of the ketoacidosis and diabetes mellitus is warranted. Assessment of serum insulin can be made, but is rarely useful as there is little else that will result in such a marked hyperglycaemia.

143 i. Calcium oxalate. Approximately 95% of nephroliths are composed of calcium-containing salts. Middle-aged and older, male small breed dogs are at risk for the development of calcium oxalate uroliths. The acidic urine favours calcium oxalate, ammonium urate and cystine urolith formation, whereas struvite forms in neutral to alkaline urine.
ii. They may form secondary to hypercalcaemia or hypercalciuresis. The latter is associated with intestinal hyperabsorption of calcium or renal tubular leak of calcium. Other potential mechanisms include hypocitric aciduria, hyperabsorption of calcium from bone and hyperoxaluria.
iii. An alkalinizing diet restricted in protein, calcium and sodium was recommended. Inducing diuresis is beneficial; many protein restricted diets induce a diuresis because of medullary washout. Dietary magnesium and phosphorus should neither be restricted nor present in excessive quantities. Avoiding foods and supplements containing vitamins C and D are beneficial because vitamin C is a precursor for oxalic acid and acidification and vitamin D promotes intestinal calcium absorption and renal excretion. If the above measures are unsuccessful, supplemental vitamin B6 may be of benefit, or treatment with hydrochlorothiazide which may lower urinary calcium excretion. Potassium citrate supplementation may help because it is alkalinizing and citrate forms a soluble complex with calcium making it unavailable for precipitation with oxalic acid.

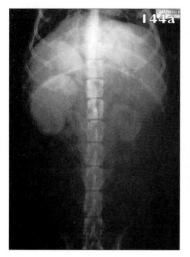
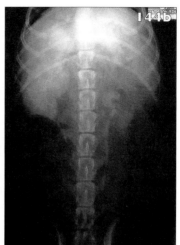

144 An 18-month-old, female Fox Terrier suffered pyrexia, depression, lethargy, vomiting and abdominal pain several days after ovariohysterectomy. Ten days following surgery the dog started to leak urine from the vulva and an acquired ectopic ureter was suspected. The dog could urinate normally and urine bacteriology confirmed a urinary tract infection. An intravenous urogram and ultrasound examination of the kidneys were performed and an acquired left ectopic ureter confirmed (144a–144c).

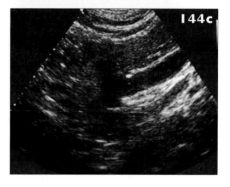

i. Describe the changes seen.
ii. What is the most likely disease process affecting the left kidney?

145 Which of these statements about hypoadrenocorticism are true and which are false?
i. Hypoadrenocorticism is primarily a disease of older female dogs (average 11 years).
ii. Aldosterone is the deficient hormone responsible for the electrolyte changes.
iii. Polyuria and polydipsia often develops in animals with hypoadrenocorticism because of a water diuresis due to renal tubular epithelial cell dysfunction.
iv. Eosinopenia and lymphocytosis occur in 80% of animals with hypoadrenocorticism.
v. Hypoglycaemia is occasionally seen in affected animals.

144 i. Different phases of an intravenous urogram are shown in **144a** and **144b**. In the nephrogram phase (**144a**) the left kidney is small and has an irregular margin compared to the right kidney. On the pyelogram (**144b**) the left ureter is distended but there is no evidence of gross dilation of the renal pelvis. There is a lucent area overlying the left kidney on both films which is gas within the descending colon. The ultrasound image of the left kidney (**144c**) reveals loss of the normal internal renal architecture and dilation of the renal pelvis and left ureter. This also confirms that the left kidney is small and irregular.

ii. The most likely disease process affecting the left kidney is pyelonephritis and obstructive nephropathy. The left ectopic ureter now opens into the vagina as well as communicating with the bladder, allowing infection to ascend the dilated ureter. Although the ureter is now patent, the history, clinical signs and radiographic findings all suggest that the left ureter was totally obstructed from the time of surgery until the urinary incontinence began.

145 i. False. Hypoadrenocorticism is characteristically a disorder of middle-aged (mean age 4–4.5 years) female dogs.
ii. True.
iii. False. Polyuria and polydipsia develop in animals with hypoadrenocorticism due to a solute diuresis. The lack of aldosterone results in reduced absorption of sodium and chloride and water, and the hyponatraemia results in a loss of the medullary concentrating gradient.
iv. False. Eosinopenia and lymphocytosis are only recognized in 10% of animals with hypoadrenocorticism.
v. True.

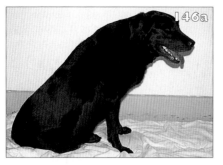
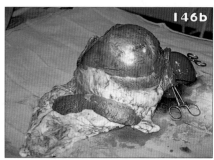

146 An eight and a half-year-old, female Labrador Retriever presents for evaluation of lethargy, intermittent weakness and collapse of two weeks' duration. Her abdomen has become progressively distended and she groans when she lays down as if in discomfort (146a). Her plasma liver enzyme activities are increased (ALT 2,849 u/l, ALP 2,959 u/l) and her blood glucose is low (2.3 mmol/l). On physical examination her abdomen is taut and a large firm mass is palpable in the cranial abdomen. Radiographically the normal caudal border of the liver is indistinct and extends beyond the costochondral junction. The stomach and loops of small intestine are displaced caudally and dorsally indicating a massive hepatomegaly. Abdominal exploratory surgery is performed and the left lateral lobe of the liver is found to be consumed with an irregular mass (146b). The remainder of the liver parenchyma is normal in appearance; no other masses are observed in the abdomen. Thoracic radiographs show no evidence of metastatic disease.

i. What are your differential diagnoses for the liver mass?
ii. What are the possible reasons for the episodes of collapse?
iii. Can you explain the laboratory finding of hypoglycaemia?

147 i. Identify the parasite in this faecal smear (147) from a puppy with chronic diarrhoea.
ii. In what other form is this parasite sometimes seen?
iii. What drugs are available for its treatment?

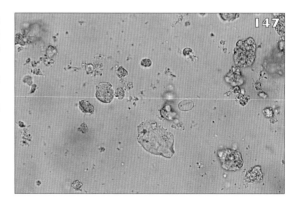

146 i. Given the size of this tumour and the absence of other masses, this is a primary tumour of liver origin. Liver tumours may be benign or malignant, and histopathology is necessary to distinguish between the two cell types. Benign hepatocellular adenomas or haemangiomas may cause abdominal discomfort and distension due to expansion of the mass and crowding of other viscera. They may recur locally if not excised totally, whereas complete removal of the tumour may be curative. However, malignant hepatocellular carcinomas or haemangiosarcomas may not have visible metastases at the time of diagnosis, but micrometastatic disease is likely and recurrence or spread into the hepatic lymph nodes, lung or peritoneum is common. The prognosis for malignant liver tumours is poor.

ii. Collapse may have occurred due to cardiovascular, metabolic or neuromuscular disease. Cardiac dysrhythmias are a frequent occurrence in animals with tumours such as haemangiosarcomas, and syncopal episodes occur due to insufficient cerebral oxygenation. However, recovery from these episodes is usually rapid and complete. Metastatic brain disease cannot be ruled out as a possible cause of neurological disease and collapse, but the signs would more likely be progressive and one might expect to see more pronounced, persistent neurological dysfunction. Myasthenia gravis is a paraneoplastic disorder affecting the neuromuscular junction and may cause intermittent weakness. Hypoglycaemia may result in weakness and even coma and seizure activity if blood glucose concentrations are severely decreased. Another cause for collapse in this dog would be an intermittent intra-abdominal bleed from a rupture of the tumour, and acute hypotension. This hypothesis is supported by the presence of anaemia, abdominal distension, the presence of blood in the abdomen and the need for several days to recover while blood is being reabsorbed by the peritoneum.

iii. Hypoglycaemia is a reported abnormality in some animals with both benign and malignant liver tumours, and can result in clinical signs of lethargy and collapse. The pathogenesis of decreased blood glucose concentrations is not completely clear, but may occur due to the tumour's increased uptake and utilization of glucose or the tumour itself may produce hormones with insulin-like activity.

147 i. A *Giardia* oocyst. These are best seen in zinc sulphate flotations, but multiple samples may have to be examined as excretion is intermittent.

ii. Occasionally, motile trophozoites are seen in very fresh smears, but they are easier to find in duodenal juice collected endoscopically.

iii. *Giardia* has been treated historically with quinacrine or metronidazole. Quinacrine is not readily available and has an unpleasant taste, and so is rarely used. High doses of metronidazole (30 mg/kg p/o q12h for 5 days) can eliminate *Giardia* but this is close to the neurotoxic dose. In addition, metronidazole-resistant *Giardia* have been reported. Successful treatment with furazolidone has been reported, but its use is not licensed for small animals. Albendazole (25 mg/kg p/o q12h for 5 days) and fenbendazole (50 mg/kg p/o q24h for 3 days) are effective. They are safe and easy to administer, and have the distinct advantage of eliminating metazoan parasites as well.

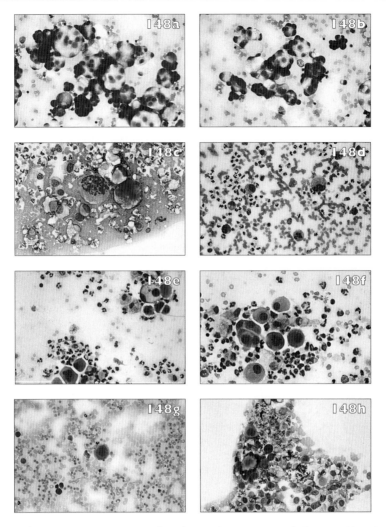

148 Cytology preparations (stained with Wright's stain) made by centrifugation of pleural and peritoneal effusions are shown (148a–148h).

148a and 148b – 11-year-old, female cat with pleural effusion.

148c and 148d – middle-aged Cocker Spaniel with pleural effusion.

148e and 148f – aged, female cat with ascites.

148g and 148h – middle-aged Lurcher with ascites.

Which photomicrographs show neoplastic effusions? On what grounds do you base the diagnosis of neoplasia and which types of neoplasms are represented? Identify the large single cells in the centre of 148c and 148g.

148 • **148a, 148b:** The cat had an intrathoracic adenocarcinoma. Note the acinar clustering of the pleomorphic neoplastic cells. Some of the cells are distended with secretion.

• **148c, 148d:** The large cell just to the left of centre in **148c** is a very large and bizarre mitotic figure. This dog also had a carcinoma. The features which differentiate this from a non-neoplastic effusion are more subtle. They include the presence of atypical mitotic figures and the degree of pleomorphism of the cells. In **148d** a trinucleate cell, a mitotic figure and four other pleomorphic cells with anisokaryosis are present.

• **148e, 148f:** This cat had an intra-abdominal carcinoma. Note the neoplastic cluster in **148f**. This cluster shows anisokaryosis, nuclear moulding and a mitotic figure.

• **148g, 148h:** The large cell in the centre of **148g** is a binucleate mesothelial cell. Note the eosinophilic corona around the periphery. This effusion developed secondarily to restrictive pericarditis. The large basophilic cells present in this effusion are reactive mesothelial cells and macrophages.

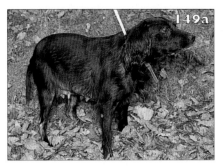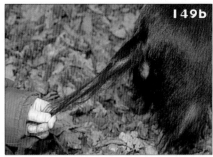

149 This eight-year-old, neutered female dog (**149a**) presented with a four-month history of lethargy, bilaterally symmetric non-pruritic alopecia and a rat-tail (**149b**).
i. What is the most likely diagnosis?
ii. Is there an age or breed predisposition for this condition?
iii. How would you confirm a diagnosis?
iv. What is the recommended treatment?

150 A five-year-old, neutered female domestic shorthair cat has been vomiting for six days. Results of laboratory evaluation are shown.
i. What is your interpretation of the azotaemia (pre-renal, renal, postrenal), and what diagnosis would you consider?
ii. What is the mechanism for hypercalcaemia in this disease?

Urea (mmol/l)	27
Creatinine (µmol/l)	221
Sodium (mmol/l)	136
Potassium (mmol/l)	7.1
Total CO_2 (mmol/l)	14
Calcium (mmol/l)	3.1
Phosphorus (mmol/l)	2.1
Serum amylase (u/l)	1,200
Urine SG	1.017
Urine protein	Negative
Urine casts	Few, granular

151 True or false?
i. The serum half-life of feline ALP activity is one-eighth of canine ALP or six hours.
ii. ALP production and release in cats is not induced by corticosteroids and anti-convulsant therapy as in dogs.
iii. The presence of bilirubin in feline urine is always abnormal and precedes hyperbilirubinaemia.
iv. Increased serum GGT activity parallels ALP activity in the cat, as it is associated with impaired biliary flow and has a bone isoenzyme.
v. The liver is responsible for producing all of the feline coagulation factors, therefore cats with severe liver failure are prone to bleeding tendencies.

149 i. Hypothyroidism. Many endocrine diseases result in a non-pruritic alopecia but the development of a rat-tail appears to be a more common feature of hypothyroidism. Lethargy is also a relatively common sign of hypothyroidism. Primary hypothyroidism due to lymphocytic thyroiditis or follicular atrophy is the most likely cause in an adult dog.
ii. There appears to be a predisposition for middle-aged to older large breeds, particularly neutered females.
iii. Thyroid stimulating hormone (TSH) test/combined total T4 and endogenous TSH. Hypercholesterolaemia, mild normochromic normocytic anaemia and a low serum total T4 concentration support a diagnosis of hypothyroidism but can also occur in a variety of other diseases. Confirmation of a diagnosis has relied on demonstrating minimal or no increase in serum total T4 concentrations after administration of TSH or thyrotropin releasing hormone (TRH). Assaying endogenous canine TSH obviates the need for TSH stimulation. In primary hypothyroidism, circulating TSH concentrations are high in the face of a low total T4 concentration.
iv. Sodium levothyroxine normalizes both circulating T4 and T3 concentrations. The initial dose is 20–22 mg/kg p/o q12–24h with further dose adjustments based on clinical response and post-pill testing.

150 i. Azotaemia with inappropriately dilute urine is consistent with renal azotaemia. However, the Na:K ratio is 19:1 which is consistent with hypoadrenocorticism. Hypoadrenocorticism often results in azotaemia with dilute urine and may be mistaken for primary renal failure. An ACTH stimulation test revealed non-detectable plasma cortisol concentrations before and after intramuscular administration of ACTH. Therefore, hypoadrenocorticism was the diagnosis.
ii. Hypercalcaemia occurs in approximately one third of cases with hypoadrenocorticism and is most likely to result from excessive renal tubular absorption of calcium.

151 i. True.
ii. True.
iii. True.
iv. False. GGT does not have a bone isoenzyme, but the serum GGT elevation typically does parallel the rise in ALP activity in most hepatic diseases except in feline hepatic lipidosis.
v. False. The liver does produce most of the coagulation factors, but not all of them. Those factors that do not rely on synthesis by the liver include factor VIII, von Willebrand's factor, which is produced by endothelial cells, and calcium. It is true that cats are prone to bleeding tendencies in states of liver failure due to the lack of production of essential coagulation factors by the liver.

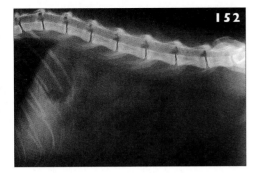

Sodium (mmol/l)	142
Potassium (mmol/l)	3.9
Calcium (mmol/l)	2.6
Glucose (mmol/l)	6.9
Urea (mmol/l)	16.5
Creatinine (μmol/l)	220
Phosphate (mmol/l)	1.7
ALT (u/l)	60
ALP (u/l)	300
Bile acids (μmol/l)	10
Bilirubin μmol/l)	15.8
Amylase (u/l)	1,900
Lipase (u/l)	300
Total protein (g/l)	75
Albumin (g/l)	30
Globulin (g/l)	45
TLI (μg/l)	120

152 A four-year-old, neutered male domestic shorthair cat presented with episodic vomiting (bilious material and food) and depression for the past few months. The bouts of vomiting were becoming more frequent. Appetite was normal other than when the cat was showing signs. Drinking was unremarkable. No diarrhoea was recognized. The cat resented abdominal palpation, although whether this was due to pain was unclear. No other physical abnormalities were noted. The clinical pathology results are shown. Abdominal radiography was performed (152). Haematology showed a mild neutrophilia with a left shift. Red cell parameters were unremarkable.

i. What is your interpretation of the clinical pathology results, and what other tests might you request?
ii. What is your interpretation of the radiograph?
iii. What treatment would you recommend?

153 An eight-year-old Springer Spaniel is presented with constipation of several months' duration. Constipated faeces were palpable on rectal examination. Physical examination was otherwise unremarkable. A barium enema was given and this radiograph was obtained (153).

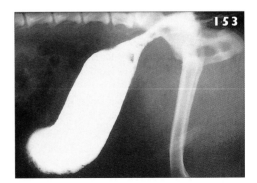

i. What is your interpretation of the radiograph?
ii. What are the causes of this condition?
iii. What treatment would you suggest?

152 i. The elevated TLI is consistent with a diagnosis of pancreatic damage, e.g. pancreatitis. Elevated amylase and lipase concentrations may also be expected with pancreatic damage, although they are often normal, and are elevated with other conditions, most notably renal failure (pre-renal or renal). The elevated ALP and normal ALT are consistent with cholestasis/hepatocyte swelling rather than ongoing hepatocellular damage, which may reflect a primary hepatopathy. However, pancreatitis can cause bile duct obstruction or hepatotoxic effects which could account for the abnormal liver parameters. There is no indication of hepatic dysfunction, although hyperbilirubinaemia is occasionally recognized with pancreatitis. The raised urea and creatinine are consistent with primary renal failure and pre-renal azotaemia. Assessment of urine SG is required to differentiate between these conditions. Hypocalcaemia is not present in this cat and, although a reported anomaly in pancreatitis cases, it is very rarely seen and is not specific for pancreatitis. Hyperglycaemia may be a feature of pancreatitis and reflects islet cell dysfunction. In the cat, hypoglycaemia appears to be a commoner finding in cases of chronic pancreatitis. The neutrophilia is consistent with pancreatitis, although in many cases haematology may be unremarkable.
ii. The abdominal radiograph was unremarkable. In acute severe pancreatitis, loss of definition in the cranial abdomen may be appreciated due to a localized peritonitis. In cases of chronic pancreatitis, plain radiography is usually unhelpful.
iii. Treatment is aimed at reducing pancreatic secretions. This can be achieved by starving the animal for a couple of days and provision of intravenous fluids. Subsequently, a low-fat, highly digestible diet is recommended.

153 i. The colon is markedly dilated along its entire length. The colonic walls are smooth but there does appear to be a narrowing of the colon at the pelvic inlet. This would be consistent with stricture formation, but may also be seen when the colon has not been adequately filled with barium, or if there is a peristaltic wave passing down the colon. After administration of more barium this narrowed area disappeared, suggesting that it was artefactual rather than due to a stricture.
ii. Megacolon is diffuse dilation of the colon with ineffective motility. It may occur secondary to mechanical (intramural/extramural masses, foreign bodies) or functional (hypokalaemia or hypothyroidism) obstructions which prevent defecation for prolonged periods. In this case no underlying disorder was found.
iii. Treatment is often unsuccessful. High-fibre diets which bulk up faeces may be useful where there is some residual motor function. An increase in colonic volume is more likely to stimulate peristalsis than an empty colon. In some cases, highly digestible low-fibre diets, which produce little residue, are more helpful. Laxatives such as liquid paraffin or docusate sodium are required to ensure the faeces remain soft. Where medical therapy fails, subtotal colectomy is the only remaining option.

154 This liver biopsy (154, Masson trichrome stain, ×42 original magnification) was obtained surgically in a six-year-old, female crossbreed dog presented with decreased appetite, weight loss and occasional vomiting of six weeks' duration. Clinical pathology revealed hyperglobulinaemia (47 g/l), hypoalbuminaemia (22 g/l) and elevated liver enzymes

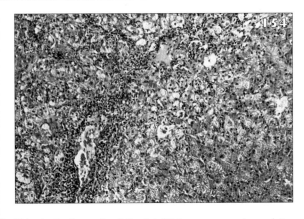

(ALT 918 u/l, ALP 645 u/l). Urinalysis showed a SG of 1.026, trace protein and 2+ bilirubin. Fasting serum bile acids were 225 µmol/l. Abdominal radiography revealed reduced liver size.

i. What are your comments on the liver biopsy.

ii. Does the liver biopsy explain the clinical signs and laboratory abnormalities?

155 Laboratory evaluation of a seven-year-old, male Australian Shepherd Dog with a two-month history of polyuria and polydipsia is shown. Urine cytology revealed moderate numbers of struvite crystals only.

i. What is your interpretation of the laboratory evaluation?

ii. What is your diagnosis?

iii. Contrast the different types of this syndrome?

Albumin (g/l)	32
ALP (u/l)	50
ALT (u/l)	40
Total protein (g/l)	72
Urea (mmol/l)	8.9
Creatinine (µmol/l)	62
Glucose (mmol/l)	5.6
Sodium (mmol/l)	150
Potassium (mmol/l)	3.8
Chloride (mmol/l)	132
Calcium (mmol/l)	2.6
Phosphorus (mmol/l)	1.7
Total CO_2 (mEq/l)	7
Anion gap (mEq/l)	22
Urinalysis:	
SG	1.011
pH	7.5
Glucose, ketones, bilirubin, occult blood, protein	Negative

154 i. The biopsy shows severe chronic hepatitis, characterized by marked periportal accumulation of mononuclear inflammatory cells which are invading the hepatic lobule and infiltrating the hepatic parenchyma. The severity and invasive nature of the infiltrate is similar to that seen in human chronic active hepatitis, which has an autoimmune aetiology.

ii. Yes. Clinical signs of liver disease are often vague and non-specific, as in this case, and laboratory analysis is therefore essential. In this dog it showed marked liver enzyme elevation indicative of hepatocellular damage (ALT) and cholestasis (ALP). Low serum albumin may be due to reduced production by a chronically diseased liver, since there is no evidence for albumin loss via the kidneys or gut. Hyperglobulinaemia is common in acquired liver disease and reflects reduced Kupffer cell function, induction of acute phase proteins and development of autoantibodies. High fasting serum bile acid concentrations confirm the presence of a hepatic problem and are an indication to perform liver biopsy.

155 i. The presence of hyperchloraemic metabolic acidosis (elevated chloride, low total CO_2 and a normal anion gap) implies loss of bicarbonate from the body. Because the urine pH is inappropriately alkaline with the metabolic acidosis, the loss of bicarbonate is probably occurring in the urine.

ii. These laboratory findings are most consistent with renal tubular acidosis (RTA).

iii. Type I RTA (distal RTA) results from impaired excretion of hydrogen ions into the distal nephron. Type II RTA (proximal RTA) results from an impaired reabsorption of bicarbonate ions from the proximal tubular lumen. Type IV RTA is due to aldosterone deficiency or resistance resulting in decreased hydrogen ion secretion by the distal nephron and in hyperkalaemia which impairs ammonium ion production and excretion.

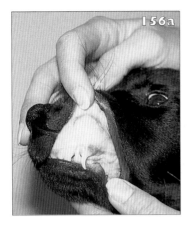 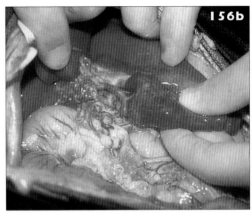

156 This three-month-old, entire female Flat Coated Retriever presented with a gradual onset of abdominal distension, dark, tarry stools and progressive lethargy over the past month. On physical examination she was thin, with a markedly distended abdomen and fluid wave on ballottement. Her mucous membranes were pale (156a) and she was depressed and reluctant to walk. Abdominal exploratory surgery revealed a small liver with a mass of large, tortuous vessels visible (156b). A portovenogram demonstrated an enlarged vessel with a palpable thrill. This was thought to be an anomalous connection between the hepatic vein and the portal vein.
i. Can you explain the pathophysiology of the ascitic fluid formation and anaemia based on the imaging studies?
ii. What is the prognosis, and what therapy can be offered?

157 A ten-year-old, entire male Boxer (157) is presented with polyuria and polydipsia of several months' duration. The dog is nocturic. The dog drinks in excess of 150 ml/kg/day and will attempt to drink water out of sinks and the toilet at any opportunity. He is in a lean body condition, but has a good appetite and is not losing weight. No other abnormalities are reported and physical examination is unremarkable. You suspect diabetes insipidus.
i. How might you proceed to confirm your diagnosis?
ii. How would you treat diabetes insipidus?

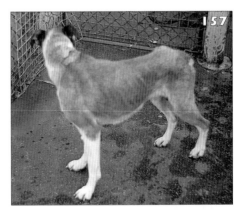

156 i. The finding of an intrahepatic arteriovenous anastomosis is compatible with the presence of portal hypertension and the formation of ascites due to increased hydrostatic pressure and leakage of hepatic lymph into the peritoneal space. GI bleeding, evidenced by the melenic stools, and resultant anaemia are often the result of gastroduodenal ulcerations, which may occur with portal hypertension, and coagulopathies due to decreased factor production by the liver.

ii. The prognosis for this congenital defect is, unfortunately, very poor. Palliative therapy with fresh whole blood, gastric protectants and diuretics may help to improve the immediate distress, but is unlikely to have any long-lasting benefits.

157 i. A full serum biochemistry screen is indicated initially to rule out other causes of PU/PD (such as renal disease, hepatic disease, electrolyte disorders, etc.) prior to performing a water deprivation test. Urinalysis is required to check urine SG (dilute urine would be expected with diabetes insipidus). Urine sediment should be inactive with a trace to no proteinuria. Haematology is usually normal in dogs with diabetes insipidus.

A water deprivation test is indicated if no other metabolic cause for the clinical signs is evident. The modified water deprivation test is indicated. This involves an abrupt deprivation of water followed by assessing response to vasopressin. Following water deprivation, urine SG and body weight are assessed every two hours until the urine concentrates or 5% of body weight is lost. If there is a failure to concentrate urine, DDAVP (desmopressin acetate) (2 μg i/v) is administered and urine SG monitored hourly for up to four hours when the urine should have concentrated. A failure to respond to water deprivation but a response to DDAVP is consistent with central diabetes insipidus. A failure to respond to DDAVP is consistent with a form of nephrogenic diabetes insipidus.

Misdiagnoses may occur if medullary washout is present. This could be ruled out prior to the water deprivation test by slightly restricting water intake and adding salt to the food for five days prior to testing.

ii. Diabetes insipidus is treated by replacing antidiuretic hormone (ADH). This is achieved by administering DDAVP (a synthetic analogue of ADH). The intranasal preparation should be used for long-term use. It may be administered by placing drops into the nose or onto the conjunctivae. It is not essential to treat provided a dog has free access to water.

158 This dark field micro-scopy photomicrograph (**158**) was taken of urine obtained from a four-year-old, unvac-cinated male Boxer who was pyrexic, anorexic and began vomiting three days prior to presentation after swimming in a stagnant farm pond. On clin-ical examination the dog was jaundiced, mildly dehydrated and depressed. Haematological findings included a neutrophil-

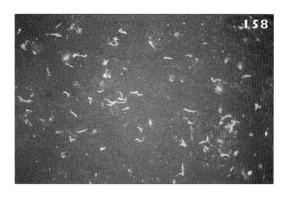

ia (21.3 × 10^9/l) with a mild left shift (3.2 × 10^9/l band cells), and a thrombocytopenia (8.7 × 10^9/l).

i. Can you identify the shape of the organism demonstrated by this technique?
ii. When would this particular test be indicated?
iii. If this test was not available, how else could you arrive at this diagnosis?
iv. Would appropriate vaccination prophylactics have protected this dog from disease?

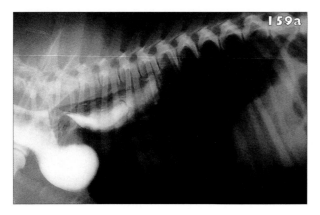

159 An adult, small breed dog presented with vague signs of apparent pain after eat-ing, occasionally accompanied by retching and regurgitation immediately after eat-ing. The dog was keen to eat and at all other times was normal. He exercised well and was active. A thoracic radiograph was taken after administration of barium (**159a**).

i. What is your diagnosis?
ii. What is the cause of the problem?
iii. How would you treat this condition?

158 i. The organisms viewed are spiral in shape and are *Leptospira* spp.

ii. Dark field microscopy (DFM) is a technique used for rapid identification of leptospires within urine of infected dogs. As leptospires are not readily isolated, DFM provides a rapid means of diagnosis in animals that are suspected of being infected based on signs of acute renal or hepatic failure in an endemic area.

iii. Culture of *Leptospira* organisms requires special growth media and they commonly prove difficult to isolate. Antibody titres are commonly used to demonstrate infection. Since *Leptospira* bacterins are a part of most routine vaccination protocols, most animals will have a low baseline antibody titre. Paired serum antibody concentrations will demonstrate increasing titres and, hence, active disease. Serum titres should be evaluated in the acute stage upon presentation; a convalescent titre is obtained 2–4 weeks later and this should show a four-fold rise in titres in actively infected animals.

iv. Routine vaccinations contain the two main serovars of *Leptospira*, *L. canicola* and *L. icterohaemorrhagiae*. Immunization is effective in reducing the severity and prevalence of infection, but does not prevent the carrier state. There is little to no crossover in immunity with different serovars such as *L. pomona* or *L. grippotyphosa*, which also result in clinical renal and hepatic failure in infected animals. Animals in endemic areas should receive frequent vaccinations.

159 i. The radiograph shows a barium-filled outpouching from the oesophagus and dilatation cranial to the lesion. The diagnosis is an oesophageal diverticulum.

ii. Acquired oesophageal diverticula are classified as pulsion or traction forms. The former result from increased

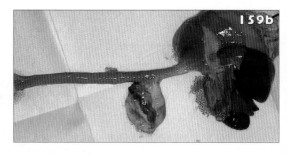

intraluminal pressure or from herniation of mucosa through a disruption in the muscular layer of the oesophageal wall. They do not contain layers of muscle wall and most commonly arise secondary to an oesophageal foreign body. Traction diverticula occur secondarily to perioesophageal inflammation in which all layers of the oesophageal wall are pulled away from the lumen to form an evagination.

A developmental redundancy of oesophageal tissue seen at the thoracic inlet may be present in young animals, particularly brachycephalic breeds. This pouch reduces in size as the neck is extended and tends to disappear as the dog matures.

iii. Surgical excision (**159b**). The owners of this dog elected for euthanasia.

160 This mesenteric portogram (**160**) was obtained in a one-year-old, male Cairn Terrier with a history of intermittent diarrhoea and vomiting, inappetence and failure to gain weight. More recently the owners had noticed aimless wandering and disorientation following feeding. Physical examination revealed a thin, depressed dog. The most notable finding in blood tests was

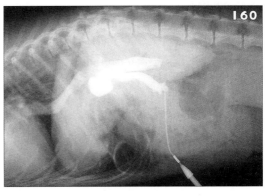

markedly elevated serum bile acid concentrations (pre-prandial 336 µmol/l, postprandial 521 µmol/l). Abdominal radiography showed a small liver.

i. Why and how is mesenteric portography performed?
ii. What is your diagnosis?
iii. Does this explain the clinical signs?
iv. What is the treatment of choice for this dog?

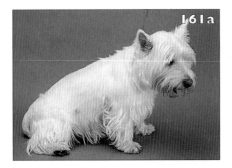
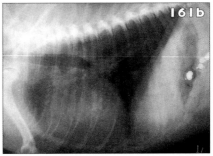

161 A two-year-old, male West Highland White Terrier has a six-month history of intermittent vomiting and diarrhoea (**161a**). When afflicted with GI signs the dog frequently eats grass. Recently the dog has become very lethargic when exercised and occasionally coughs. Haematological examination reveals an eosinophilia (6.3 × 10⁹/l) and basophilia (0.9 ×10⁹/l). There is no murmur but chest radiographs show significant right heart enlargement and a patchy bronchointerstitial pattern in the lung (**161b**). Barium impregnated polyspheres (BIPS) are still present in the stomach eight hours after administration, and follow-up radiographs show delayed gastric emptying. Faecal examination reveals the presence of *Giardia* oocysts and some larvae.

i. What parasites might this dog have?
ii. How did the dog acquire the infections?
iii. How would you treat them?

160 i. Mesenteric portography is performed to document the presence and location of a portosystemic vascular anomaly. A loop of jejunum is isolated through a small ventral midline laparotomy. An over-the-needle catheter is inserted and secured in place, and a water-soluble contrast medium (e.g. Urografin 370 or Omnipaque 350) (1 ml/kg body weight) is injected as a bolus. A single lateral radiograph is taken as the final millilitre of contrast medium is injected, and another injection is made in order to obtain a ventrodorsal view. Congenital portosystemic shunts may also be demonstrated ultrasonographically, but portography is often still performed to confirm the location and determine the potential for surgery.

ii. The portogram shows a single extrahepatic portosystemic shunt.

iii. Yes. The vague multisystem clinical signs are typical of what can be seen in dogs with a congenital portosystemic shunt. With the exception of stunted growth or failure to gain weight, clinical findings can be highly variable. Neurological signs resulting from hepatic encephalopathy occur commonly and may be prominent following ingestion of a high-protein meal. Signs typically wax and wane. Routine laboratory evaluation can be unremarkable but may reveal erythrocyte microcytosis, variable liver enzyme elevation, low blood urea, hypocholesterolaemia and/or hypoglycaemia. The most important finding is marked increase in serum bile acid concentrations (especially postprandial). Blood ammonia concentration may be increased, but due to problems in obtaining a reliable assay this is less commonly measured in practice. Liver size is often reduced, since the liver atrophies due to the lack of hepatotrophic factors present in portal blood.

iv. Partial or total ligation of the aberrant vessel. Extrahepatic shunts are more accessible for ligation than intrahepatic shunts, but improved surgical technique has led to a greater success rate for the ligation of intrahepatic shunts as well. Shunt surgery requires experience and expertise, and is best carried out in a referral situation. Most animals improve markedly after surgery. Medical management of hepatic encephalopathy, using lactulose, oral antibiotics and a low-protein diet, is essential before surgery and should also continue postoperatively as regeneration of liver tissue requires several months.

161 i. The dog does have *Giardia* infection which is probably responsible for the GI signs, but the intense eosinophilia and basophilia is not typical of simple giardiasis. The presence of larvae in the faeces, in association with coughing, is consistent with *Oslerus osleri* (*Filaroides osleri*) or *Angiostrongylus vasorum* infection. The mild right heart failure, radiographic pulmonary changes and characteristic larval morphology are consistent with angiostrongylosis.

ii. The long history of GI signs suggests that the dog's original problem was the *Giardia* infection. Delayed gastric emptying is probably associated with intestinal inflammation. *Giardia* oocysts are usually acquired by ingestion of faecally contaminated water. The consequent GI disease caused the dog to eat grass and, in doing so, it inadvertently ate the molluscs that are the intermediate host of *Angiostrongylus*.

iii. Both *Giardia* and *Angiostrongylus* can be treated with fenbendazole.

162 A six-year-old crossbreed dog is presented for profuse vomiting and depression four days after having ripped a carpet to shreds. A string found wrapped around the base of the tongue extended down the oesophagus. Endoscopically a piece of carpet was seen to be attached to the string and other string was seen to pass through the pylorus. The string around the tongue in this dog was cut and a large mat of carpet retrieved via a

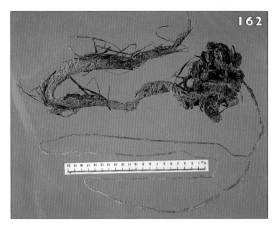

gastrotomy (162). The strings passing down the small intestine were also pulled out through the stomach. The dog made a full recovery.

What potential complications occur in animals that have a linear foreign body, and how are such complications managed?

163 A two-year-old male Labrador is presented collapsed with pale mucous membranes, bradycardia, inappetence for 24 hours and anuria for 12 hours. He has a history of vague lethargy, intermittent vomiting and diarrhoea. You suspect hypoadrenocorticism and take blood samples to make the diagnosis. Complete the table below with the values of the parameters you might expect if this dog has hypoadrenocorticism.

	Result	(Normal)
ALT (u/l)		(<80)
ALP (u/l)		(<100)
Bile acids (μmol/l)		(<15)
Glucose (mmol/l)		(3.5–5.5)
Urea (mmol/l)		(<9)
Creatinine (μmol/l)		(<110)
Calcium (mmol/l)		(2–3)
Phosphate (mmol/l)		(0.9–2.3)
Sodium (mmol/l)		(140–153)
Potassium (mmol/l)		(3.8–5.3)
Basal cortisol (nmol/l)		(<260)
Post-ACTH cortisol (nmol/l)		(<660)

162 • Vomiting and dehydration, which must be managed by intravenous fluid therapy. Antiemetics such as metoclopramide are contraindicated if there is intestinal obstruction, as they increase the impaction of the foreign body and may cause a perforation to develop.
• Removal of a long string may require multiple enterotomies. However, a technique of attaching the string to a rubber catheter through a proximal enterotomy and then 'milking' the catheter along the intestine out through the anus has been described.
• Perforation of the intestine frequently occurs at numerous sites as the string acts as a 'cheese wire' cutting through the intestinal wall where it bunches. Careful examination of the whole length of the intestine and repair of every hole is mandatory. If perforation has occurred, abdominal lavage with copious volumes of sterile saline and aggressive antibiotic therapy (such as intravenous clavulanate-potentiated amoxycillin and metronidazole or gentamicin) are indicated. Drainage is required in severe cases of peritoneal contamination and septic peritonitis; closed drains (e.g. Penrose drains) are ineffective in the peritoneal cavity and open peritoneal drainage is required.

163 Elevations in urea, creatinine and potassium concentrations, and a low sodium concentration would be expected. Hypocalcaemia and hypoglycaemia are variable features. ALT, ALP, bile acids and phosphate would be expected to be normal. A low basal cortisol value which fails to rise significantly following administration of ACTH is required to make the diagnosis of hypoadrenocorticism. The values obtained in this dog were:

	Result	(Normal)
ALT (u/l)	90	(<80)
ALP (u/l)	120	(<100)
Bile acids (μmol/l)	4.8	(<15)
Glucose (mmol/l)	4.2	(3.5–5.5)
Urea (mmol/l)	67	(<9)
Creatinine (μmol/l)	1,200	(<110)
Calcium (mmol/l)	1.8	(2–3)
Phosphate (mmol/l)	1.0	(0.9–2.3)
Sodium (mmol/l)	122	(140–153)
Potassium (mmol/l)	7.1	(3.8–5.3)
Basal cortisol (nmol/l)	<12.5	(<260)
Post-ACTH cortisol (nmol/l)	<12.5	(<660)

164 A 12-year-old, neutered male, 28 kg Irish Setter began vomiting 24 hours prior to presenting in a collapsed state. The owners describe the vomitus as bile-coloured with flecks of coffee ground-type material present. On physical examination the dog was pale, depressed, tachycardic (150 bpm) and had weak peripheral pulses. PCV was 0.17 l/l with no regenerative response apparent. A transfusion of fresh whole blood was administered and an endoscopic examination of the stomach was performed (164).

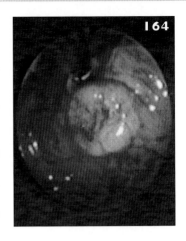

i. Describe what you see, and give a list of differential diagnoses.
ii. How will you proceed to reach a definitive diagnosis?

165 A photomicrograph of a cytology preparation from the centrifuged sediment of a pleural effusion from a young adult cat (165). It is stained with Wright's stain.

What is the diagnosis?

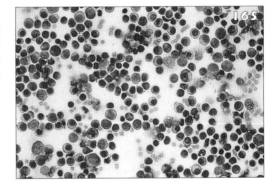

166 An Irish Setter with chronic intermittent diarrhoea and weight loss is diagnosed as having gluten-sensitive enteropathy (166).
i. What is gluten?
ii. How can this dog be treated?
iii. Is the Irish Setter the only breed that can suffer from gluten sensitivity?

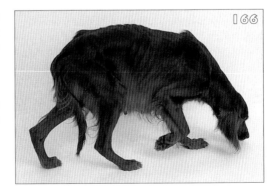

164 i. There is a raised, rounded lesion adjacent to the cardia which appears to be supported by a stalk of tissue and has a central mucosal defect or ulcer. This ulcer is likely to be responsible for the vomiting, rapid blood loss and collapsed state of the dog on admission. The anaemia is likely to be non-regenerative because of the rapidity of the blood loss and lack of time for the bone marrow to respond. Causes of gastric ulceration include: administration of drugs such as NSAIDs or steroids which alter the mucous barrier and gastric blood flow; repeated exposure to allergens or toxins; severe systemic illness and resulting hyperacidity such as liver and renal failure; neurological disease; or gastric ischaemia associated with trauma, shock or hypoadrenocorticism, primary neoplastic disease or paraneoplastic disorders such as mast cell degranulation or hypergastrinaemia due to a gastrinoma. Pertinent to this dog's history was the administration of phenylbutazone (200 mg every other day) for the past four weeks for treatment of arthritis.

ii. This dog was apparently healthy prior to the acute onset of vomiting, but subclinical systemic disorders should be ruled out by performing a complete biochemical profile, blood count and urinalysis. Serum gastrin assays may help rule out gastrin-producing pancreatic tumours which may be small and otherwise not visible on routine imaging studies. Other than the anaemia, all other laboratory parameters were normal for this dog. Barium contrast studies may demonstrate ulcers but may not reveal subtle mucosal lesions. Endoscopic examination allows visualization of the ulcer and enables mucosal biopsies to be obtained to differentiate an inflammatory lesion from neoplasia. Care must be taken not to disturb the central area of the lesion when obtaining biopsies as this may induce further bleeding. Histopathology was consistent with inflammation or reactive hyperplasia rather than neoplasia.

165 Intrathoracic malignant lymphoma. This is quite a pleomorphic population of lymphoblasts and lymphocytes. Unlike lymph node aspirates, in which the presence of lymphoblasts in modest numbers is a normal finding, the appearance of lymphoblasts in an effusion is nearly always diagnostic of malignant lymphoma.

166 i. Gluten is the alcohol-soluble protein found in wheat and related cereals, namely barley, rye and oats.

ii. Gluten-sensitive enteropathy can be successfully managed by feeding a gluten-free diet. Rice and maize (corn) are gluten free and are suitable cereal sources that can be fed; wheat, barley, rye and oats should be avoided. Mashed potato is an alternative source of starch. Gluten sensitivity has been definitively demonstrated in Irish Setters by biopsy-proven remission on a gluten-free diet and relapse on gluten challenge. However, such strict criteria are unlikely to be applied in the practice setting.

iii. Although it has yet to be proven beyond doubt in other breeds, it would be surprising if no other dog breeds were susceptible. Indeed, gluten sensitivity is already suspected in Soft-coated Wheaten Terriers and Samoyeds.

167 A photomicrograph of an aspirate from a retrobulbar mass is shown (**167**). It is stained with Wright's stain.
i. Describe the cytological appearance of the aspirate.
ii. What is the diagnosis?

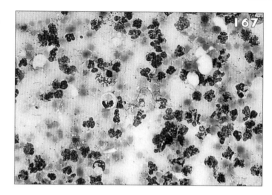

168 This hepatic ultrasonogram (**168**) was obtained in a 12-year-old cat with a two-month history of intermittent anorexia, vomiting and jaundice. The cat responded transiently to fluid therapy and antibiotics, but the signs would recur. The cat was mildly jaundiced and in moderate body condition. Abdominal radiographs showed mild hepatomegaly. Haematology was normal. Serum biochemistry revealed hyperbilirubinaemia (35 μmol/l), elevated liver enzymes (ALT 345 u/l, ALP 765 u/l) and hypercholesterolaemia (11.2 mmol/l).

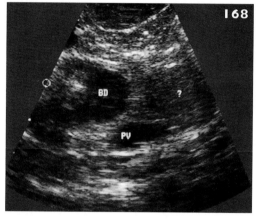

i. What are your differential diagnoses?
ii. What do you see on the hepatic ultrasound picture?
iii. How would you proceed to obtain a definitive diagnosis?

169 A four-year-old Dobermann is presented with weight gain, bilaterally symmetrical non-pruritic alopecia, lethargy and inappetence. You suspect hypothyroidism.
i. What clinical biochemistry/haematology features might you expect in routine tests, and why do they develop?
ii. How would you confirm the diagnosis?
iii. What are the causes of hypothyroidism?

167 i. This is a good example of degenerate neutrophils with both extracellular and intracellular bacteria which are a mixture of rods, cocci and chains of rods.
ii. Retrobulbar abscess.

168 i. The cat has hepatobiliary jaundice, with both cholestatic and hepatocellular involvement. Liver enzymes in the cat have a short half-life, and this degree of enzyme elevation is very significant. The high cholesterol concentration could indicate extrahepatic bile duct obstruction, but this finding is not as helpful in the cat as in the dog since in the cat many conditions tend to be accompanied by hypercholesterolaemia. Similarly, most liver diseases in the cat result in hepatomegaly. Considerations in this cat would be: cholangiohepatitis, extrahepatic bile duct obstruction, neoplasia, hepatic lipidosis, FIP (less likely) and other miscellaneous causes (such as hepatic amyloidosis).
ii. Ultrasonography shows marked dilation of the bile duct (BD), almost to the diameter of the portal vein (PV). Caudal of the liver, a lucent mass (?) is observed in the area of the pancreas. Therefore, this cat has extrahepatic bile duct obstruction possibly due to a pancreatic lesion.
iii. Extrahepatic bile duct obstruction is an indication for exploratory laparotomy. Bile duct obstruction in the cat is often due to neoplasia (especially pancreatic adenocarcinoma) compressing the common bile duct, as was the case in this cat. Other causes include bile duct compression by pancreatitis, sludged bile associated with the cholangiohepatitis complex, choleliths or bile duct strictures. Surgical intervention may involve a cholecystotomy and bile cultures in case of choleliths, or more radical biliary diversion procedures in case of strictures or neoplasia. Pancreatic neoplasia is usually inoperable.

169 i. Serum cholesterol is raised in 66–75% of hypothyroid dogs due to decreased lipoprotein lipolysis and a reduction of low density lipoprotein receptors. These alterations result in an increase in very low density and low density lipoproteins, i.e. hypertriglyceridaemia and hypercholesterolaemia. Where a myopathy has developed, an increase in creatine kinase activity may be seen. Other routine biochemical assays are unremarkable. Haematologically a mild non-regenerative, normochromic, normocytic anaemia may develop in 25–40% of affected dogs due to reduced RBC production
ii. Assessment of total plasma thyroxine levels may be useful. However, non-thyroidal illness will secondarily reduce plasma T4 levels. Free T4 may be assayed as an alternative as this is less susceptible to artefactual lowering. Measurement of canine thyroid stimulating hormone (TSH) in conjunction with assessment of thyroxine is more helpful as a low thyroxine but high TSH is more suggestive of hypothyroidism. With non-thyroidal disease a normal TSH value would be expected. Thyroid stimulation tests are useful, although rarely used because of the limited availability of pharmaceutical grade TSH and variable responses to thyrotropin releasing hormone (TRH).
iii. Primary hypothyroidism, the commoner form, develops due to lymphocytic thyroiditis or thyroid atrophy. Congenital hypothyroidism (thyroid agenesis, dysgenesis or dyshormonogenesis) is uncommon. Central hypothyroidism usually results from adenohypophyseal or hypothalamic neoplasia. Central congenital hypothyroidism, most often hypophyseal compression by a cystic Rathke's pouch, is rare.

170 A kitten you vaccinated two days previously has returned with upper respiratory tract (URT) signs. The owner says your vaccine made the cat sick; he is angry and is threatening to sue both you and the vaccine manufacturer. On examination you find that the kitten's tongue is ulcerated (170).

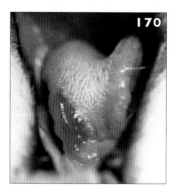

i. What do you think caused the clinical signs?
ii. How are you going to prove it?
iii. What explanations could account for the clinical signs appearing so shortly after vaccination?
iv. Which of the explanations is most likely?
v. Have you been professionally negligent?

171 A 13-year-old, neutered male Dachshund presented with acute onset seizures (1–2 minutes' duration), particularly at exercise and often immediately prior to a feed. Between fits the dog was normal. The dog was fed twice a day and had a good appetite. No other historical features were reported by the owner. Physically the dog was overweight; no other abnormalities were evident. Blood glucose was 2.4 mmol/l, calcium 2.5 mmol/l, sodium 147 mmol/l, potassium 4.6 mmol/l, urea 4.8 mmol/l, creatinine 990 µmol/l, ALP 500 u/l, ALT 200 u/l, bile acids 1.5 µmol/l. Haematology was unremarkable.

i. What diagnosis would you consider to be most likely?
ii. What further diagnostic tests would you perform?

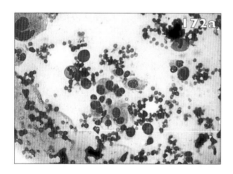
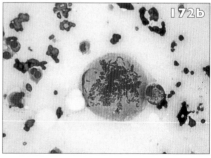

172 Two photomicrographs of an aspirate from a rapidly growing, 2 cm diameter, solid subcutaneous mass from the caudal lumbar area of a 12-year-old cat are shown (172a, 172b).

i. Describe the cytological findings in 172a.
ii. What is the structure in the centre of 172b?
iii. Is this a malignant neoplasm?

170 i. Feline calicivirus infection (FCV) (though feline poxvirus (cowpox virus) can, occasionally, also cause oral ulceration).

ii. Take a swab from the oropharynx into viral transport medium and send it to a laboratory for virus isolation. Unlike feline herpesvirus, FCV is shed continually, but most cats spontaneously recover and eliminate the virus.

iii. (a) The cat was incubating a FCV infection already; the period from infection with FCV to development of clinical signs is 2–10 days; or (b) the vaccine was aerosolized, causing URT infection by the vaccine virus; or (c) the vaccine virus had not been attenuated properly.

iv. It is most likely that the cat was already incubating FCV infection at the time of vaccination. Vaccine manufacturers have careful quality control to ensure that vaccinal viruses do not cause severe clinical signs: suspected breakdowns should be reported to the manufacturer. To demonstrate that vaccinal virus did not cause the clinical signs, the FCV isolated from the cats can be compared, by plaque-typing and cross-neutralization testing, with the isolate used in the vaccine.

v. Only if you did not give the cat a thorough clinical examination, including temperature and oral mucosa checks, before administering the vaccine. Aerosolizing the vaccine is accidental rather than negligent.

171 i. The hypoglycaemia could account for the seizures. The observation that the fits occur prior to feeding or at exercise when the blood glucose is lowest is an important factor. Idiopathic epilepsy is more likely to occur at rest than at exercise. The normal calcium provides no evidence of hypocalcaemia. Other metabolic causes which can probably be eliminated include hepatic encephalopathy, as the dog is normal between fits and the bile acids are unremarkable. Hypoglycaemia in this older animal is most likely due to an insulinoma but may also develop in end-stage hepatic failure, hypoadrenocorticism, extrapancreatic tumours, growth hormone deficiency and cortisol deficiency. Although end-stage hepatic failure is unlikely in this dog, the ALP and ALT are elevated. This may reflect a benign subclinical hepatopathy or tumour metastasis to the liver.

ii. Documentation of elevated plasma insulin and low blood glucose taken at the same time is helpful. Radiography is rarely helpful. Ultrasonographic examination of the pancreas may demonstrate the mass and it can be used to assess the liver for metastases.

172 i. The aspirate contains blood and a highly pleomorphic population of round to spindyloid cells. The neoplastic features present are anisokaryosis, variable numbers of nuclei per cell, variable size of nuclei within a multinucleate cell, mitotic figures, variable cytoplasmic basophilia, variable numbers and size of nucleoli, and nuclear moulding.

ii. An extraordinary, enormous mitotic figure.

iii. There are numerous criteria for malignancy in these photomicrographs. Cytological classification of neoplasms as malignant must always be very cautious because some benign neoplasms have numerous cytological criteria for malignancy and some malignant neoplasms appear cytologically benign. Malignancy really reflects the behaviour of a tumour rather than its appearance *per se*. This neoplasm has malignant potential.

173 While performing a post-mortem examination on a cat which had a history of weight loss and intermittent anorexia and dullness, you find this lesion in the kidney (173).
i. What are the two most likely diagnoses of the lesion?
ii. How are you going to confirm the diagnosis?
iii. What will you advise about testing the client's other two cats in each of the two conditions?

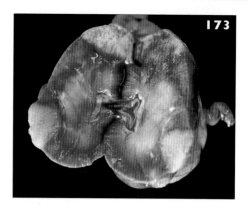

174 Match the serum biochemistry results below with the description of the animal they most likely represent, and give a short explanation of the pathogenesis for these changes or the lack thereof. For each dog there is a corresponding best matching set of values such that all choices will be used when properly matched. Choose carefully, since some animals may match two or more of the choices provided.

	Dog 1	Dog 2	Dog 3	Dog 4	Dog 5
ALP (u/l)	402	274	1,248	2,480	200
ALT (u/l)	45	68	145	1,200	586
Bile acids (mmol/l)					
– fasted	6	28	38	41	107
– postprandial	12	162	49	64	136

a. Six-month-old, male Yorkshire Terrier with a portosystemic shunt, on antibiotic and lactulose therapy, and currently behaving normally.
b. Twelve-year-old, neutered female Cocker Spaniel displaying polydipsia, polyuria, polyphagia, weight gain and abdominal distension.
c. Six-year-old, entire female Golden Retriever with acute vomiting and diarrhoea, abdominal pain and elevated plasma lipase and amylase concentrations.
d. Three-month-old, entire female Labrador; clinically normal.
e. Nine-year-old, neutered male Maltese Terrier with hepatic cirrhosis and stable clinical signs.

173 **i.** Renal lymphoma or FIP pyogranuloma. The first may be FeLV or FIV related.
ii. Histopathology.
iii. If histopathology confirms the presence of lymphoma, test the remaining two cats for FeLV and FIV for the following reasons: 85% of FeLV positive cats are dead within 3.5 years, so FeLV infection will seriously affect the cat's life expectancy; cats should not be introduced where there are FeLV or FIV infected cats; FeLV and FIV are immunosuppressive. Owners need to be alerted to the possibility that infections can be more serious in FeLV and FIV infected cats than in normal cats, so that they can seek veterinary attention earlier.

If FIP is confirmed, discuss with the owner the possibility of testing for FCoV antibodies. Since FCoV is very contagious, you would expect the two in-contact cats to be seropositive, therefore testing is not worthwhile except for obtaining an antibody titre for comparison with a second test 3–6 months later. If the immunofluorescent antibody titres have fallen to less than 10, it is safe to introduce a new cat. Some 90% of seropositive cats do not develop FIP.

174 Dog 1 – d. Alkaline phosphatase has three major isoenzymes; liver, bone and corticosteroid-induced. Young growing puppies normally have a mildly increased serum ALP activity due an increase in the bone isoenzyme.
Dog 2 – a. Animals with portosystemic shunts commonly have normal liver enzyme activities unless they have other encephalopathic or sepsis-induced liver enzyme activity. Classically these dogs have a normal to mildly increased fasted bile acid concentration which increases dramatically postprandially.
Dog 3 – b. This is a classic description of a dog with hyperadrenocorticism. The greater increase in ALP than ALT enzymatic activities is due to the corticosteroid-induced isoenzyme, and a normal to mildly increased ALT concentration is likely from hepatocellular leakage and glycogen storage in steroid hepatopathies. Mild increases in serum bile acid concentrations may occur.
Dog 4 – c. Pancreatitis should be a high consideration in this animal and these liver enzyme activities would support that diagnosis. Cholestasis resulting from a pancreatitis results in increased ALP production and, depending on the severity of inflammation, the ALT activity will increase as well but typically to a lesser extent.
Dog 5 – e. Animals with chronic, quiescent hepatic cirrhosis may have normal to mild increases in liver enzyme activities despite decreased hepatic function, as evidenced by moderate elevations in both fasted and postprandial bile acids.

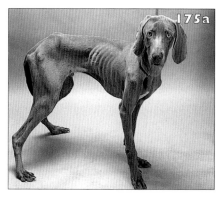
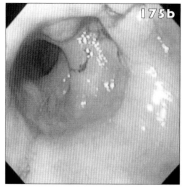

175 A ten-year-old Weimaraner is anorexic and has profuse diarrhoea and severe weight loss (**175a**). Panhypoproteinaemia plus lack of proteinuria or elevated bile acid concentrations have led to the tentative diagnosis of a protein-losing enteropathy (PLE). Endoscopically the duodenum is poorly distensible with pale, smooth and thickened mucosa (**175b**).
i. What diseases can cause a PLE?
ii. Which is most likely in this case?
iii. How would you make a diagnosis and treat this dog?

176 Your client breeds Ragdoll cats and has a recurrent problem every year with fading kittens. All the cats in the household are vaccinated against FPV, FCV, FHV and FeLV and boosters are up to date. All the cats are routinely tested negative for FIV, FeLV, FCoV antibodies and *Chlamydia*. One morning your client presents you with one dead three-week-old kitten which died suddenly overnight, and a nine-week-old kitten from another litter which was perfectly all right yesterday but is presented today collapsed, with a subnormal temperature, dehydrated and close to death.
i. The owner does not want euthanasia of the nine-week-old kitten. How are you going to treat it?
ii. What is your tentative diagnosis?
iii. How will you confirm your diagnosis?
iv. Why are littermates of affected kittens clinically healthy at present?
v. How will you protect the littermates?
vi. What advice will you give the Ragdoll breeder to prevent recurrence of this problem?

175 **i.** IBD; lymphocytic-plasmacytic enteritis (LPE); eosinophilic enteritis; granulomatous enteritis; lymphangiectasia; intestinal lymphosarcoma.

ii. The age and anorexia are typical of intestinal lymphosarcoma but severe IBD could also be the cause. The appearance of the duodenum is typical of cellular infiltration of the mucosa, but the appearance is not diagnostic of any specific disease.

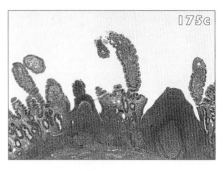

iii. Intestinal biopsy. Endoscopic biopsies can be too superficial or too distant from the primary lesion to give an accurate diagnosis. In addition, LPE can coexist with lymphosarcoma. Multiple endoscopic biopsies are more likely to give an accurate diagnosis but interpret biopsy results with caution. Full thickness surgical biopsies taken from several levels of the intestine are indicated to show malignant lymphocytes within the mucosa and infiltrating the submucosa and muscular layers (**175c**). Intestinal lymphosarcoma is poorly responsive to combination chemotherapy; patients are often severely malnourished because of the associated malabsorption and are less tolerant of chemotherapy. Thus the prognosis is guarded to grave.

176 **i.** Treat the kitten symptomatically with intravenous fluids and a heat pad.

ii. Feline parvovirus (FPV) (feline panleucopenia virus or feline infectious enteritis).

iii. Take large intestinal contents from the three-week-old kitten and faeces or rectal swabs from the living kitten to check for FPV. As FPV can pass through a cat or kitten in under 48 hours, other confirmatory tests are needed in case the result is negative. Submit duodenum, jejunum and ileum for histopathology. Take blood from the living kitten and the adults in the household for FPV serology. Antibody titres following natural exposure are much higher than in vaccinated cats.

iv. Some littermates will be protected by maternally derived antibody. The amount any kitten receives depends on the queen's antibody titre and how well the kitten sucked. Many kittens survive FPV infection and may not become clinically ill, but stress such as rehoming or intercurrent intestinal infection can push a kitten into clinical disease. This can manifest as sudden death.

v. Remove them to a clean household before their maternally derived antibody wanes. To calculate their approximate titre, take the queen's titre and halve it for every two weeks of the kitten's life.

vi. The best advice is to stop breeding kittens for a year. This will allow the amount of virus in the premises to decrease. FPV can survive for up to a year in the environment. There is no carrier state. Viral propagation depends on susceptible animals being introduced; therefore, by stopping introducing susceptible new kittens and cats or only introducing fully vaccinated cats, virus can be eliminated from an environment. Parvocidal disinfectants will help to reduce virus load, but virus will still be present in furnishings and carpet which cannot be disinfected.

177 This one-year-old, female Deerhound has been experiencing behavioural abnormalities where she intermittently appears blind, will stand and stare, or will press her head against a wall (177a). On physical examination she was in poor body condition, severely depressed, barely responsive and semi-comatose (177b).

i. What underlying disease states lead to hepatic encephalopathy?

ii. What concurrent clinical and biochemical abnormalities contribute to hepatic encephalopathy?

iii. How are you going to treat the current clinical signs?

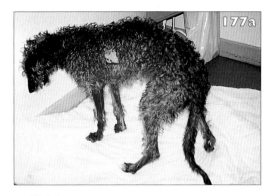

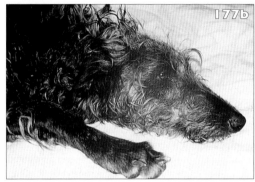

178 True or false?

i. Hepatic AST is released later and typically represents a consequence of more severe injury than do increases in serum ALT activity.

ii. With acute, severe hepatic disease, an increase in ALP precedes hyperbilirubinaemia followed by bilirubinuria.

iii. Hypercholesterolaemia occurs in liver failure due to the increased production of very low density lipoproteins (VLDLs).

iv. Since the liver is responsible for producing the majority of coagulation factors, normal screening tests such as prothrombin times (PT) and activated partial thromboplastin times (APTT) are used as sensitive indicators of normal liver function.

v. Coagulopathies due to obstructive jaundice and relative vitamin K deficiency lead to the decreased production of factors II, VII, IX and X and results in prolonged bleeding times. The administration of parenteral vitamin K may improve the PT and partial thromboplastin time (PTT) by greater than 30% within 24 hours.

177 i. Hepatic encephalopathy refers to a spectrum of neurological disorders associated with advanced liver disease. In young dogs such as this one, a congenital portocaval shunt should always be suspected, particularly considering that Deerhounds are predisposed to intrahepatic shunting. Acquired liver diseases such as acute hepatic failure of any origin, or chronic cirrhotic or fibrotic livers with secondary portosystemic shunting, can result in hepatic encephalopathy in animals of any age.

ii. Dehydration, azotaemia, alkalaemia and hypokalaemia. Therapy should be aimed at their correction. Secondary infections and constipation can lead to increased bacterial production of ammonia and GI bleeding may provide a high-protein substrate for ammonia production.

iii. The definitive treatment is surgical ligation of the shunting vessel; however, encephalopathic patients must first be managed medically:

• In acutely encephalopathic patients demonstrating signs of seizures, amaurosis and potentially coma, early intervention is needed to prevent or treat cytotoxic cerebral oedema and increased intracranial pressure. Management includes fluid therapy, enhanced oxygenation and intravenous mannitol.

• In the clinically disoriented, lethargic but otherwise stable shunt patient, a low-protein diet should be fed and antibiotic therapy with ampicillin or metronidazole should be instituted directed at decreasing the urease-producing gram-negative organisms and their production of ammonia. Lactulose is a synthetic sugar which acidifies the colonic contents, converting the freely diffusable ammonia to non-diffusable ammonium ions which become trapped within the colon and excreted in the faeces. Other benefits of lactulose therapy include a reduction in the enteric flora and the induction of an osmotic catharsis. If the patient is constipated, lactulose can be diluted in water and given as an enema. The use of prednisolone should be avoided as it contributes to protein catabolism. Gastric protectants such as sucralfate and ranitidine may be necessary in animals with liver disease, portal hypertension and GI bleeding.

178 i. True.
ii. False. Bilirubinuria precedes hyperbilirubinaemia.
iii. False. Cholesterol is synthesized in the liver from dietary and endogenous sources of lipids, and in liver failure, serum cholesterol concentrations are usually low.
iv. False. Coagulation factors may be reduced by 25–30% of normal function due to decreased production by the liver before these screening tests detect deficiencies. Therefore, although they are important in determining the consequences of liver failure, they are not very sensitive tests of liver function.
v. True.

179 Match each of the six sets of results below with the appropriate diagnosis/clinical description? Some result sets may apply to more than one diagnosis, therefore choose what you see as the best fit.

	Calcium (mmol/l)	Phosphate (mmol/l)	Parathyroid hormone - (PTH) (pmol/l)
A	1.2	3.6	<1
B	1.7	0.9	4.2
C	1.8	5.7	29
D	1.8	1.2	20
E	1.2	4.2	12
F	1.1	1.2	10

i. Ten-year-old dog presented with acute onset grand mal seizure. Prior to the fit the dog had been stiff and inappetent for a few days.

ii. Lactating bitch presented following a seizure. She whelped four weeks previously and is feeding eight pups.

iii. Dog presented with weight loss. Laboratory results: urea 6.7 mmol/l, creatinine 100 µmol/l, albumin 15 g/l, globulin 35 g/l, cholesterol 10.2 mmol/l, urine protein:creatinine ratio 5.8. You suspect a protein-losing nephropathy.

iv. Two-year-old dog presented several hours after the ingestion of antifreeze containing ethylene glycol. The dog is depressed, acidotic and hyperkalaemic.

v. Nine-year-old dog presented with chronic PU/PD of several months' duration, anorexia, weight loss, vomiting, urine SG 1.014, blood urea 34 mmol/l, creatinine 400 µmol/l.

vi. Nine-month-old crossbreed dog presented with a pathological fracture of the right tibia. The dog was fed exclusively an all-meat diet.

180 This lateral abdominal radiograph (**180**) is of a four-year-old, unilateral cryptorchid male dog exhibiting bilaterally symmetrical non-pruritic alopecia, gynaecomastia and attractiveness to male dogs.

i. What is your radiographic interpretation?

ii. What is the likely diagnosis?

iii. What other clinical signs might you expect?

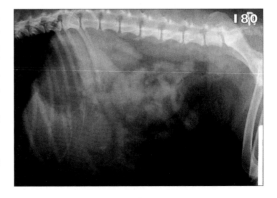

179 i. A. This dog had primary hypoparathyroidism. The clinical signs can be very vague. The finding of a low calcium, low PTH but high phosphate value is very suggestive of primary hypoparathyroidism.

ii. F. Marked hypocalcaemia may develop in lactating bitches resulting in seizures. Phosphate and PTH values are usually unremarkable, although PTH may be elevated.

iii. B. The description is consistent with a protein-losing nephropathy. Hypo-albuminaemia may result in a mild hypocalcaemia as calcium is protein bound. Plasma ionized calcium would be normal.

iv. E. Ethylene glycol will cause severe hyperphosphataemia and a concomitant fall in calcium following acute ingestion. Subsequently, calcium chelation by metabolites of ethylene glycol also results in hypocalcaemia. Severe renal damage, acidosis and hyper-kalaemia are also seen. The PTH should be normal following acute intoxication, but possibly raised once renal failure results.

v. C. The history is typical of chronic renal failure. In such cases, serum calcium may be low, normal or high, but phosphate is usually elevated. With the development of renal secondary hyperparathyroidism, PTH is also increased.

vi. D. The history is typical of secondary nutritional hyperparathyroidism. In such cases the PTH is driven high by the imbalanced calcium:phosphorus ratio associated with consumption of a meat only diet. Calcium and phosphate may be normal or low.

180 i. A round soft tissue mass is seen in the mid-abdominal region. Displacement of the intestines ventrally suggests that this mass may be of retroperitoneal origin.

ii. Testicular tumour, most likely a Sertoli-cell tumour. This diagnosis is supported by the finding of a large intra-abdominal mass in this cryptorchid dog, because retained testicles are at greatest risk for the development of tumours, particularly Sertoli-cell tumours. The dog is exhibiting typical clinical signs of the male feminizing syndrome as a result of either increased production of oestrogens by testicular tumour cells, increased conversion of testosterone and androstenedione to oestrogens by testicular tissue or peripheral tissues, or an abnormality in the balance of the sex hormones as a result of decreased androgen production in the face of normal oestrogen production. In dogs this syndrome is most commonly associated with Sertoli-cell tumours.

iii. Other possible clinical signs include anaemia, hyperpigmentation, a pendulous penile sheath and standing in a female posture to urinate.

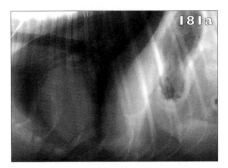
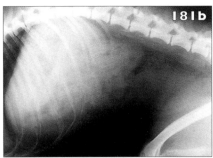

181 Lateral view abdominal radiographs of two dogs are shown (181a – dog 1; 181b – dog 2). The serum biochemical results for these two dogs are shown.

i. Describe the radiographic abnormalities common to both dogs.
ii. What are the differential diagnoses of these findings?
iii. Are further diagnostic tests indicated, and if yes, which ones?

	Dog 1	Dog 2
Total protein (g/l)	51	62
Globulin (g/l)	29	32
Albumin (g/l)	21	30
Total bilirubin (µmol/l)	183.4	3.6
Urea (mmol/l)	3.2	5.5
ALT (u/l)	2,255	54
ALP (u/l)	873	145
Cholesterol (mmol/l)	2.33	6.9
Bile acids (µmol/l)	67.6	8

182 A five-month-old, male Dalmatian is presented because of difficulty chewing food. He had been purchased at three months of age and had always drunk large quantities of water. The confirmation of his head had always been different from his littermates (182a). Radiographs of the skull were obtained (182b).

i. What is your diagnosis?
ii. How can this condition be treated?
iii. What is the prognosis?

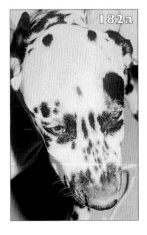
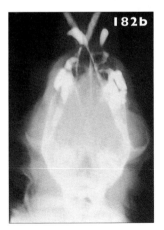

181 i. The normal radiographic position of the liver is just caudal to the diaphragm with its caudal edges bordering upon the stomach, the right kidney and the proximal duodenum. The caudoventral tip of the liver is normally blunted and lies just caudal to the costochondral cartilages. The stomach is typically angled with the fundus or ventral most region directed caudally. This can vary amongst breeds, particularly in deep chested dogs. In both lateral views the caudal most tip of the liver does not reach the costochondral junction and the angle of the stomach is such that the fundus is directed cranially indicating possible microhepatica. A ventrodorsal view would also be indicated to confirm the cranial position of the stomach and other abdominal viscera.

ii. Microhepatica is associated with congenital portosystemic shunts, hepatic cirrhosis, hepatic fibrosis or potentially severe hypotension. In rare instances an otherwise normal liver may appear small due to a partial intrathoracic location as in animals with pleuroperitoneal or pericardioperitoneal diaphragmatic hernias.

iii. The signalment, history and clinical signs are very important in assessing the patient's clinical picture, interpreting the results and directing future diagnostics.

Dog 1 is a six-year-old, male crossbreed which has been anorexic, lethargic and vomiting for two weeks and has biochemical parameters indicative of hepatic damage. Further investigation such as liver function tests, postprandial bile acids and a hepatic biopsy is warranted.

Dog 2 is an eight-year-old, female Irish Setter with palpable splenomegaly and anaemia. Her biochemical profile is normal and her signs are not consistent with hepatic disease; the size of her liver may be normal for her size and breed. Therefore, a liver biopsy would not be indicated at this time.

182 i. Fibrous osteodystrophy, probably secondary to chronic renal failure.

ii. Reduce serum phosphorus concentration utilizing dietary restriction and possibly oral intestinal phosphate binding drugs, which include aluminium hydroxide, carbonate and oxide (30–90 mg/kg/day), or calcium acetate (60–90 mg/kg q24h), carbonate and citrate (90–150 mg/kg q24h). Use calcium-containing phosphorus-binding agents with caution if administering vitamin D concurrently. Vitamin D administration in conjunction with proportional reduction in phosphate intake has been shown to limit the development of renal secondary hyperparathyroidism and its associated skeletal abnormalities, although hypercalcaemia may develop. Calcitrol (1.5–3.5 ng/kg p/o q24h on an empty stomach) is the recommended form of vitamin D supplementation as it does not require renal activation. Monitor serum calcium, phosphate and creatinine concentrations regularly.

iii. Poor.

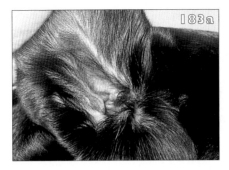

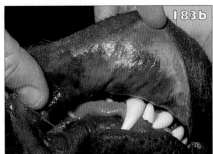

183 An eight-year-old Labrador has a two-week history of erythematous skin and mucous membranes (183a, 183b) and marked pruritus. One day prior to presentation the dog begins to vomit. He is depressed and has a painful swollen abdomen. Radiographs reveal free intraperitoneal gas and a moderate abdominal effusion. Abdominocentesis produces a bile stained exudate containing neutro-

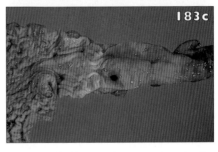

phils and engulfed bacteria. Exploratory laparotomy finds a perforating ulcer in the proximal duodenum (183c).
i. What is the significance of free intraperitoneal gas?
ii. What are the causes of GI perforation in dogs?
iii. Which of these is the most likely cause in this dog?
iv. What medical treatment is available for the treatment of gastroduodenal ulcers before perforation occurs?

184 An unvaccinated eight-month-old Dobermann is presented with acute onset depression, tachypnoea, tachycardia, jaundice and vomiting. You suspect leptospirosis.
i. How would you confirm the diagnosis?
ii. What therapy would you recommend?
iii. What are the commonest leptospiral serovars to affect dogs?
iv. How common is leptospirosis in cats?

183 i. Assuming the body wall has not been breached (e.g. a laparotomy has not been performed, no gun-shot wound, etc.), free intraperitoneal gas is indicative of a rupture of an intra-abdominal viscus and is an indication for exploratory laparotomy. Small volumes of gas are easiest to visualize between the liver and root of the diaphragm.

ii. A number of factors such as uraemia, endotoxaemia, hypovolaemia/ischaemia and steroid administration predispose to erosions/ulceration. Drugs, inflammation or neoplasia can cause damage directly, and any damage is potentiated by secretion of excess gastric acid. In order of likelihood, the causes of gastroduodenal perforation in dogs are:

- NSAID administration.
- Local neoplasia (e.g. gastric carcinoma).
- Liver disease.
- Foreign body.
- External trauma (either directly damaging the gut or interrupting the blood supply).
- Mast cell tumour.
- Gastrinoma/apudoma (Zollinger-Ellison syndrome).

iii. The history of pruritus and skin erythema are suggestive of a mast cell tumour. The tumour releases histamine, which not only affects skin but also stimulates excessive gastric acid secretion, which in turn may result in gastric or duodenal ulceration/perforation. This dog had systemic mastocytosis – large numbers of mast cells in the peripheral blood. Systemic mastocytosis, as in this case, is generally unresponsive to treatment and therefore euthanasia was carried out.

iv. Ulcer prevention is important in dogs receiving prednisolone in the treatment of local mast cell tumours, as the steroid delays epithelial turnover and predisposes to ulceration. Reducing acid secretion by histamine antagonists such as cimetidine, ranitidine or famotidine is indicated. Proton pump inhibitors (e.g. omeprazole) are more effective at inhibiting acid secretion. Any erosions can be protected by administration of sucralfate which binds to damaged tissue and prevents further acid-induced damage.

184 i. Urine/blood culture/examination for leptospires. The organism is labile and samples must be processed rapidly. Examination of a fresh wet preparation of urine under dark field microscopy may demonstrate the presence of the organism. The organism is difficult to culture. Serological assessment of paired samples at 0, 2 and occasionally 4 weeks should show a fourfold rise in titre following acute infection. Serum biochemistry is indicated to assess for hepatic/renal disease and haematology is useful in demonstrating whether a haemolytic process is present.

ii. Fluid therapy (lactated Ringer's solution or 0.9% saline) to maintain renal function as acute renal failure may develop. Penicillin/streptomycin or tetracycline for controlling and eliminating leptospires. Isolate from other dogs and prevent human infection as the organism is a zoonotic.

iii. The organisms which infect animals are serovars of *Leptospira interrogans*. The best recognized serovars are *L. icterohaemorrhagiae*, *L. canicola* and *L. grippotyphosa*.

iv. Cats have an inherent resistance to leptospires and rarely develop leptospirosis.

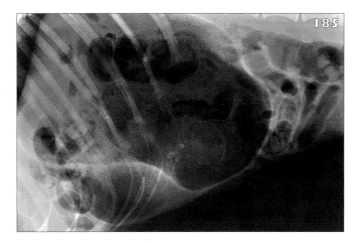

185 A six-year-old, neutered male Cocker Spaniel presents for intermittent abdominal distension associated with pain, lethargy and inappetence. The owner reports that the abdomen will distend acutely after feeding and remain so for several hours. An abdominal radiograph was taken during an episode of bloating (185).
i. What are your radiographic findings?
ii. What predisposing factors may result in gastric distension?
iii. What therapy would you recommend?

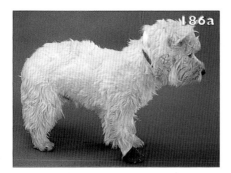
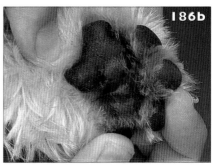

186 A two-year-old West Highland White Terrier has chronic diarrhoea, weight loss (186a) and interdigital dermatitis (186b).
i. Name two diseases that may be associated with both GI signs and pedal pruritus.
ii. How would you treat them?

185 i. There is severe gaseous dilatation of the stomach and small intestines. The axis of the stomach is displaced caudally with the antrum at the level of the 5th lumbar vertebra. The orientation of the stomach does not indicate volvulus and there are no apparent obstructing lesions. Faeces are visible in the descending colon but the rest of the intestine appears empty.

ii. Gastric distension may result from delayed gastric emptying, increased gaseous production or aerophagia. Delayed gastric motility may be a result of nervous inhibition by stress, trauma or pain. Metabolic disorders such as hypokalaemia, acidosis, uraemia or hepatic encephalopathy may cause gastric retention. Drug therapy with anticholinergics or narcotic analgesics will delay gastric emptying. Chronic obstruction may lead to distension and hypomotility of the stomach. Inflammatory lesions, such as gastritis, ulcers or infections with *Helicobacter* spp. or parvovirus, affect gastric motility adversely. Idiopathic delayed gastric emptying is a diagnosis of exclusion.

iii. Rule out the above underlying predisposing factors and correct any abnormalities found. If no organic disease is identified, feed small amounts of a semi-liquid, low-protein, low-fat diet at frequent intervals to allow rapid emptying. If diet alone is inadequate, drug therapies to increase gastric motility may be utilized. Metoclopramide (0.2–0.5 mg/kg q8h) increases the amplitude and frequency of antral contractions, inhibits relaxation of the fundus and thereby promotes gastric emptying. Erythromycin at ineffective antimicrobial doses (0.5–1.0 mg/kg q8h) most closely mimics the stimulatory effect of the GI hormone motilin, and cisapride (0.1–0.5 mg/kg q8–12h) promotes gastric emptying through activation of neuronal serotonergic and other receptors.

186 i. • *Uncinaria stenocephala* infection. This is usually associated with poor kennel hygiene; larvae gain access between the toes, causing an interdigital dermatitis and a parasitic enteritis.
• Food allergy. Concurrent pedal pruritus and diarrhoea have been reported as manifestations of suspected food allergy. Pruritus and secondary lesions of self-trauma, particularly affecting the feet and ears but with no specific pattern of distribution, are the most commonly seen dermatological manifestations of food allergy. However, other causes of pruritus, such as fleas and atopy, are much more common.

ii. Fenbendazole and nitroscanate are effective in eliminating *Uncinaria stenocephala*. Repeat treatment at three week intervals may be necessary to eliminate new adult worms as the larvae emerge from their tissue migration. Improved kennel hygiene is also required to prevent reinfection. Food allergy is treated by feeding novel dietary protein sources.

187 This ultrasound picture (187) was obtained in a two-year-old, neutered female Persian shorthair cat with a history of variable appetite, weight loss and progressive abdominal enlargement of three months' duration. On physical examination the cat was thin and had marked ascites. Haematology was unremarkable. A serum biochemical profile was normal apart from hyperglobulinaemia (globulin 46 g/l, albumin 32 g/l)

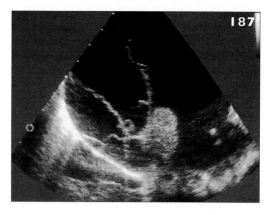

and mild ALP elevation (99 u/l). Fasting serum bile acids were 35 μmol/l. Abdominocentesis yielded light-yellow clear fluid with total protein 42 g/l and nucleated cell count 0.5×10^9/l; cytology revealed a mixture of lymphocytes, neutrophils, macrophages and occasional erythrocytes.

i. Classify the abdominal fluid. What are your differential diagnoses?
ii. How does the ultrasonogram relate to the clinicopathological findings?
iii. What further tests would you perform to obtain a diagnosis?

188 The feline coronavirus (FCoV) antibody titres of a household of cats in your care are shown below:

	Jan 95	Apr 95	Jul 95	Oct 95	Feb 96	Apr 96	Jul 96
A	320	20	20	20	0	0	0
B	20	20	20	20	10	10	0
C	320	80	160	160	160	40	20
D	640	160	>1280	1280	1280	640	640
E	80	40	80	80	80	80	80
F	320	80	80	40	20	10	0
G	160	80	320	320	320	20	0

i. What clinical signs would have alerted you to the presence of FCoV in this household, so that testing was initiated?
ii. Queen G was pregnant in July 95. What advice will you have given to the owner to prevent the kittens becoming infected with FCoV?
iii. These cats are obviously eliminating FCoV infection (their antibody titres are falling to zero). What might the owner have done to aid the elimination of FCoV from his cats?

187 i. The fluid is a modified transudate but with a high protein content approaching that of an exudate. This type of high-protein ascites can be found in cats with either lymphocytic cholangiohepatitis or FIP. Ascites is a common feature of severe chronic liver disease in the dog but not in the cat, possibly because cats with liver disease rarely develop portal hypertension. An exception is the high-protein ascites which specifically occurs in cats with lymphocytic cholangitis. Its aetiology is unclear.

ii. The ultrasonogram shows abdominal fluid accumulation and a small irregular liver with attached fibrin strands. Small liver size is suggestive of cirrhosis rather than FIP. Cirrhosis is rare in the cat but may occur as the end stage of cholangiohepatitis. Serum biochemistry in this patient shows few abnormalities indicative of liver disease, but this is not uncommon in biochemically quiescent liver diseases such as cirrhosis. Marked hyperglobulinaemia may be seen in both cholangiohepatitis and FIP. Fasting serum bile acids are only mildly increased in this patient, illustrating the need for a two-hour postprandial sample to further assess liver function. Postprandial bile acid concentrations are typically markedly abnormal in animals with cirrhosis.

iii. Liver biopsy is necessary for definitive diagnosis and prognosis. Wedge biopsy may be safer because of the risk of severe coagulopathies in end-stage liver disease, due to either disseminated intravascular coagulation and/or decreased production of clotting factors. This cat had biliary cirrhosis.

188 i. • Feline infectious peritonitis. FIP occurs most frequently in kittens which have been sold out of a household, since stress may precipitate the development of the disease.

• Diarrhoea or uneven litter size in kittens and/or transient or chronic diarrhoea in the adult cats.

ii. Kittens are protected from FCoV infection by maternally derived antibody until they are 5–6 weeks old. Kittens should be kept with their queens in isolation from other cats from birth. At 5–6 weeks of age they should be weaned and isolated from all other litters and cats, including their mother, until they are sold. They should be tested for FCoV antibodies at over ten weeks of age; before ten weeks, not all infected kittens have seroconverted.

iii. Seronegative cats should be separated from seropositive cats to prevent their reinfection. It also helps if cats are kept individually or in stable groups of up to two to three.

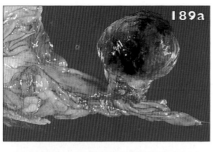
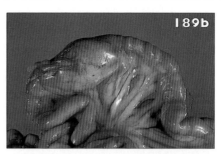
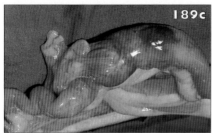
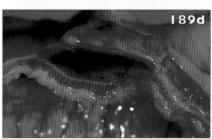

189 Abdominal masses are found in or associated with the intestine in three eight-year-old German Shepherd Dogs. In no dog is there macroscopic evidence of metastatic spread. What is the likely diagnosis in each case?

a. An incidental finding at postmortem examination of a dog with no GI signs that died of dilated cardiomyopathy. The mass appears encapsulated and is arising from the serosal surface of the ileum (**189a**).

b. A cylindrical mass within the wall of the mid-jejunum of a dog with intermittent vomiting, diarrhoea, melena and poor appetite. There is also evidence of a microcytic anaemia. On cut surface the mass is infiltrating the whole wall and the luminal surface is ulcerated (**189b**).

c. A cylindrical mass within the wall of the mid-jejunum of a dog with chronic intermittent vomiting (**189c**). Areas of haemorrhage are visible on the serosal surface and there are some adhesions to other bowel loops (**189d**). Blood-filled spaces are obvious on cut surface.

190 Which of these statements about diabetes mellitus are true and which are false?
i. Obesity causes an irreversible insulin resistance.
ii. Diabetes mellitus is more likely to develop during dioestrus in the bitch than at any other part of the reproductive cycle.
iii. Protamine zinc insulin has a duration of activity of 12 hours in dogs.
iv. When treating a dog with diabetic ketoacidosis, soluble insulin should be administered intramuscularly hourly.
v. Low-fibre diets are recommended for animals with diabetes mellitus.

189 In all three dogs the gross appearance and associated signs are suggestive of certain diagnoses, but potentially they could be associated with either a benign or malignant process. Thus biopsy would be needed to reach a definitive diagnosis in each case.

a. Leiomyoma. The lack of clinical signs associated with this mass, and its muscular attachment, make a leiomyoma most likely. These benign tumours arise from the intestinal smooth muscle and can form isolated masses. More typically they arise within the intestinal wall, where they may cause a partial or complete obstruction and, if their luminal surface ulcerates, signs of melena and anaemia may develop. Leiomyosarcomas are very rare and are unlikely to have such a circumscribed appearance.

b. Adenocarcinoma. Rectal adenocarcinomas are more common in dogs than small intestinal carcinomas, in contrast to the relative incidence in cats. Small intestinal adenocarcinomas may cause vomiting and diarrhoea because of partial or complete obstruction. If the mucosa is ulcerated, overt melena can be seen, but if bleeding is more subtle and prolonged, a microcytic iron-deficiency anaemia can develop. An isolated intestinal lymphoma would be the most likely differential diagnosis in this case, but occasionally granulomas or transmural inflammation (perhaps associated with a foreign body) have a similar appearance.

c. Intestinal haematoma. The gross appearance on cut surface was suggestive of haemangiosarcoma, although the intestine is an unusual place for metastatic spread and a primary splenic mass was not present. Histological examination revealed no evidence of a malignancy. The final diagnosis was a submucosal haematoma. Intestinal haematomas are very rarely reported in the veterinary literature and their cause is unknown. External abdominal trauma or temporary luminal obstruction with a foreign body that eventually passes, but causes intestinal wall damage, seem most likely. This dog showed no further signs after resection of the affected loop of bowel.

190 i. False. Obesity impairs glucose tolerance by down-regulating insulin receptors, which impairs receptor binding affinity for insulin and causes postreceptor defects. These effects are reversible if the obesity is managed.

ii. True.

iii. False. Protamine zinc insulin has a duration of activity in most dogs of 24 hours.

iv. True.

v. False. High-fibre diets are recommended as they result in a reduction of the postprandial hyperglycaemia.

191 An aged, overweight female Labrador presents two months after a season with a one-week history of occasional vomiting, lethargy, inappetence and, in the owner's opinion, being 'mildly off colour'. Physical examination is unremarkable and abdominal palpation impossible. Your X-ray machine has insufficient penetration for a diagnostic abdominal radiograph so you decide to take a sample for a haematological profile because you are concerned about the possibility of pyometra. Your in-house haematology analyser gives the results shown.

WBCs (× 10⁹/l)	46
PCV (l/l)	0.29
Platelets (× 10⁹/l)	95
Granulocytes (× 10⁹/l)	41.9
Lymphocytes/monocytes (×10⁹/l)	4.14

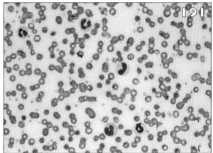

i. How would you interpret these results?
ii. Why is morphological examination of a blood film necessary for further management of this case?
  You elect to examine a blood film (**191**).
iii. Identify the white blood cells present.
iv. What is their significance?
v. Can you identify any features suggesting neutrophil toxicity?
vi. Why is the presence or absence of toxicity important?

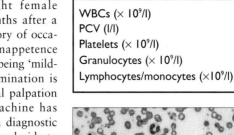

192 A seven-year-old, entire male Shih Tzu presented for evaluation of severe weight loss and chronic, progressive, vomiting occurring 1–3 times daily over the past 12 months. A barium series revealed delayed gastric emptying and retention of food in the stomach 24 hours after a meal. The endoscopic appearance of this dog's pyloric outflow tract is shown (**192**).
i. What is your diagnosis?
ii. What treatment will you recommend?

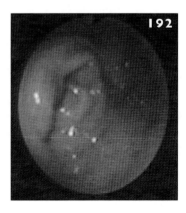

191 i. The WBC count is markedly elevated. However, most in-house analysers based on QBC principles cannot measure WBC counts greater than $30 \times 10^9/l$ with accuracy, so the value recorded in this dog could be anything above 30. The leucocytosis is due to elevated granulocytes, but their stage of maturity is unknown and thus could be a leukaemoid response (granulocyte response to an infectious stimulus) or a granulocytic leukaemia. The PCV suggests a mild degree of anaemia which could be regenerative or non-regenerative. The platelet count appears reduced, but platelet clumping, a common finding in canine and feline blood samples, can cause erroneous counts on all automated analysers; the count should be checked by film examination. The lymphocyte/monocyte count is unremarkable but could be masking a monocytosis or the presence of atypical lymphocytes, lymphoblasts or monocytes.
ii. For the reasons outlined above it would be inadvisable to make a tentative diagnosis of pyometra and elect for surgery based on this information alone.
iii. There are two bands, two metamyelocytes and a neutrophil.
iv. These immature forms suggest a marked left shift consistent with a response to infection or sepsis. These cells could also be seen in a chronic granulocytic leukaemia.
v. Toxic change is a subtle finding in canine and feline neutrophils. It is manifest as a rather foamy cytoplasm with scattered light granulation and the presence of Dohle bodies (round basophilic intracytoplasmic bodies). The magnification of this film (×60) is probably insufficient to rule out toxic changes with confidence.
vi. Toxic changes would be strongly suggestive of an infectious process in this case and would provide some basis for the discrimination between granulocytic leukaemia and a leukaemoid response.

192 i. The appearance of enlarged mucosal folds that surround and obstruct the pyloric canal is consistent with chronic hypertrophic pyloric gastropathy (CHPG). Mucosal biopsies should be obtained to distinguish this disease from similarly appearing polyps, or gastric or duodenal neoplasia. CHPG is an acquired lesion and is typically seen in older small breed dogs. The aetiology is unknown, but the condition is thought to result from chronic excessive hormonal trophic stimulation.
ii. In mild cases of CHPG, medical management with small, frequent, highly digestible moist meals may be palliative. Additionally, histamine blockers to control gastric acidity and prokinetic drugs to increase gastric motility may be beneficial in the unobstructed dog. However, when the pylorus is obstructed, as in this dog, surgical treatment is necessary to remove the excess tissue and normalize gastric emptying. Surgical procedures include mucosal resection, various forms of pyloroplasty, and gastroduodenostomy depending on the severity of the lesions.

193 This five-year-old, neutered female domestic shorthair cat (**193a**) presented with lethargy, weight loss and intermittent vomiting of one months' duration. The cat had shown similar signs during the past year but these had resolved spontaneously within a week. This time signs had persisted and become more severe. Haematology was normal. A serum biochemical profile revealed hyperglobulinaemia (globulin 56 g/l, albumin 30 g/l), hyperbilirubinaemia (69 µmol/l) and elevated liver enzymes (ALT 308 u/l, ALP 806 u/l). Abdominal radiographs showed mild hepatomegaly and ultrasonography revealed a diffuse mottled pattern with normal bile ducts.

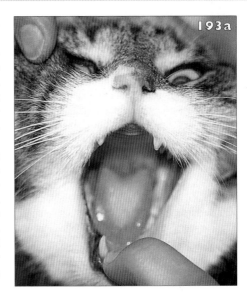

i. What are your differential diagnoses?
ii. How would you come as non-invasively as possible to a definitive diagnosis?
iii. How would you treat this cat?

194 You examine an 11-year-old, neutered male Beagle for vomiting of four days' duration. Results of laboratory evaluation are shown.
i. What is your interpretation of the azotaemia: pre-renal, renal or postrenal?
ii. What is the explanation for the hyperamylasaemia?

Urea (mmol/l)	74
Creatinine (µmol/l)	1,432
Sodium (mmol/l)	143
Potassium (mmol/l)	3.5
Total CO_2 (mmol/l)	11
Calcium (mmol/l)	2.3
Phosphorus (mmol/l)	3.9
Serum amylase (u/l)	2,400
Urine SG	1.010
Urine protein	Negative
Urine casts	Negative

193 i. Icteric primary liver diseases in the cat include the cholangiohepatitis complex, infectious disorders (including FIP), cholelithiasis, hepatobiliary neoplasia, toxic and drug-induced hepatopathies, and idiopathic hepatic lipidosis. Cholangiohepatitis complex occurs most commonly and often has vague intermittent signs, as in this cat. Cats with idiopathic lipidosis are totally anorexic, which is not the case here. FIP-associated liver disease is usually a terminal event and the animal will appear iller. Cholelithiasis and neoplasia were not identified on imaging. Several systemic infections and metabolic illnesses, such as sepsis, diabetes mellitus, hyperthyroidism, myeloproliferative disorders and hypoxia, may lead to secondary hepatic involvement and abnormal liver tests. They are less likely in this case, based on history and laboratory tests. Hyperthyroidism may cause elevated liver enzymes but rarely causes jaundice.

ii. Retinal examination may show a chorioretinitis, which may be found with FeLV or FIP. The cat should be tested for FeLV and FIV, and *Toxoplasma* serology considered. Fine-needle aspiration for cytology may be useful since the liver is diffusely enlarged; it is of most value in lymphosarcoma and hepatic lipidosis. Distinguishing between hepatocellular and obstructive biliary tract disease via ultrasonography helps to decide whether to biopsy the liver percutaneously, which is least traumatic, or whether to proceed with exploratory laparotomy and surgical biopsy, which can allow for possible surgical correction of an obstruction. Percutaneous biopsy under ultrasonographic guidance is preferred in this case. Biopsies should be submitted for histopathology and cultured aerobically and anaerobically. Coagulation status should be assessed before biopsy, especially if this is to be done blindly. Since cats with icteric liver disease often have significant cholestasis and vitamin K malabsorption, it is advisable to pretreat with vitamin K1 (5 mg/cat s/c or i/m q12h) prior to biopsy.

iii. Supportive treatment with intravenous fluids and vitamin B supplementation is indicated pending biopsy results. Ursodeoxycholic acid (15 mg/kg q24h) has hepatoprotective and choleretic effects. It is important to maintain nutrition and, if the cat is not eating, hand feeding or provision of nutritional support via nasal feeding or PEG tubes should be considered. Biopsy in this cat showed portal lymphocytic infiltrates consistent with lymphocytic cholangiohepatitis (193b). The cat was treated with prednisolone (2 mg/kg p/o q12h), which was gradually tapered off over two months, and ursodeoxycholic acid (15 mg/kg q24h). He responded well initially but relapsed when therapy was discontinued, and is maintained on 5 mg prednisolone daily.

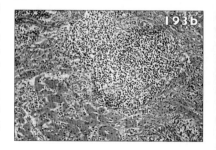

194 i. Primary renal failure. Azotaemia is present with inappropriately dilute urine (isosthenuria).

ii. Serum amylase and lipase activities are often increased with primary renal failure because they are excreted renally. With a decrease in glomerular filtration rate, amylase and lipase are retained.

195 A four-year-old, neutered female domestic shorthair cat is seen for persistent diarrhoea of four months' duration and intermittent vomiting. The appetite has not changed markedly but there has been notable weight loss. Defecation occurs once or twice daily and the diarrhoea varies in consistency from watery to semi-formed. Occasionally, mucus is present and an associated dyschezia. Abdominal palpation reveals subjectively thickened intestinal loops; the gross appearance of per-oral duodenoscopy is shown (195).

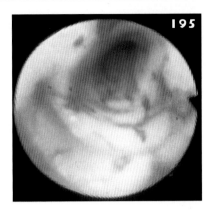

i. How would you characterize the diarrhoea?
ii. What changes can be seen on duodenoscopy, and what differentials would you consider?
   Pinch biopsies from the duodenal mucosa reveal a heavy infiltrate of lymphocytes and plasmacytes in the submucosa, with no evidence of neoplasia.
iii. What is your diagnosis?
iv. How would you manage this case?

196 An ultrasound image of the left kidney of a 12-year-old, neutered male Tonkinese cat with a history of chronic intermittent vomiting (196).

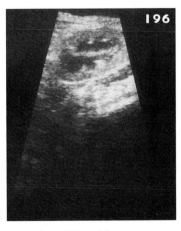

i. What is your diagnosis?
ii. In a normal glomerulus, above what size are molecules not filtered? In addition to size, what other factors influence glomerular filtration of a compound?
iii. List five functions of a nephron.
iv. A 10 kg dog was evaluated for renal failure. What laboratory methods may be used to evaluate the dog's glomerular filtration rate (GFR)?
   The following values were obtained during a 24 hour urine collection:
Volume of urine = 500 ml.
Urine creatinine concentration of the mixed 24 hour sample = 144 mg/dl.
Serum creatinine concentration at midpoint of collection = 1.5 mg/dl.
v. What is the GFR using endogenous creatinine clearance?

195 i. The diarrhoea has features of small and large intestinal disease. Small intestinal disease is indicated by the presence of weight loss, the normal frequency of defecation and the watery consistency of the faeces at times. Large intestinal disease is indicated by the dyschezia and the mucus present in the faeces. The indications are that there is a disease process affecting both large and small intestine.

ii. Duodenoscopy shows a loss of the normal 'velvety' appearance to the small intestinal mucosa and areas of marked erythema and haemorrhage. The major differential diagnoses in this case would be inflammatory bowel disease (IBD), neoplasia and duodenal ulceration.

iii. The histological description is characteristic of lymphocytic-plasmacytic IBD, the commonest form of IBD seen in cats. Clinical signs vary but usually involve one or more of vomiting, weight loss, diarrhoea and colitis. Causes of IBD include infectious or parasitic agents, or dietary hypersensitivity, and these should be excluded prior to initiating symptomatic therapy. In many cases no cause is determined and the term idiopathic IBD is used.

iv. If dietary hypersensitivity is suspected, feeding a restricted diet (single novel protein source such as venison) is recommended, but a good response to dietary modification alone is uncommon in cats. Control is usually attempted with immunosuppressive doses of prednisolone (1–3 mg/kg p/o q12h initially) but response to therapy is variable. Where improvement is seen, the dose of steroid is tapered gradually, switching to alternate day dosage if possible. If the response is poor, additional immunosuppressive drugs may have to be added to the regime, e.g. azathioprine (0.5 mg/kg p/o q48h). Metronidazole is sometimes used in addition to prednisolone therapy. Although there is little rationale for its use as an antibiotic, as feline IBD is very rarely associated with small intestinal bacterial overgrowth, it is thought to have some immune-modulating effects, and may be beneficial for this reason.

196 i. Ultrasonographically, the kidney appears normal.

ii. 68,000 daltons. Other factors include size, charge, blood pressure, blood volume and colloidal osmotic pressure.

iii. Filtration, secretion, absorption, hormone production, hormone degradation.

iv. Blood urea concentration; serum creatinine concentration; endogenous creatinine clearance; exogenous creatinine clearance; ^{14}C inulin clearance; ^{3}H-tetraethylammonium clearance; ^{125}I-iothalamate; $^{99m}Technetium$-diethylenetriaminopenta-acetic acid (DTPA).

v. GFR = clearance (ml/kg/min) = $U_x \times V/P_x \times$ time of collection $\times$ weight;
where U_x = the concentration of analyte X in a timed urine sample and P_x = the concentration of analyte X in serum or plasma at the midpoint of the timed collection.

In this case GFR = urine creatinine $\times$ volume serum creatinine $\times$ time $\times$ weight = (144 mg/dl $\times$ 500 ml)/1.5 mg/dl $\times$ 1,440 minutes $\times$ 10 kg = 3.33 ml/min/kg. (Reference range = 2–5 ml/min/kg)

Normal reference laboratory values for dogs and cats and Conversion Factors for converting SI Units to Old Units.

Haematology

	SI Units (dog)	SI Units (cat)	Con. factor	Old Units (dog)	Old Units (cat)
PCV	0.37–0.55 l/l	0.27–0.5 l/l	100	37–55 %	27–50 %
Hb	120–180 g/l	90–170 g/l	0.1	12–18 g/dl	9–17 g/dl
RBCs	$5.0–8.5 \times 10^{12}$/l	$5.5–10 \times 10^{12}$/l	1	$5.0–8.5 \times 10^{6}$/µl	$5.5–10 \times 10^{6}$/µl
MCV	60–77 fl	40–55 fl	1	60–77 mm³	40–55 mm³
MCHC	310–340 g/l	310–340 g/l	0.1	31–34 %	31–34 %
Reticulocytes	<1 %	<1 %	1	<1 %	<1 %
Reticulocytes	$20–80 \times 10^{9}$/l	$20–60 \times 10^{9}$/l	1	$20–80 \times 10^{3}$/µl	$20–60 \times 10^{3}$/µl
Platelets	$150–400 \times 10^{9}$/l	$150–400 \times 10^{9}$/l	1	$150–400 \times 10^{3}$/µl	$150–400 \times 10^{3}$/µl
nRBCs	0 %	0 %	1	0 %	0 %
WBCs	$6–15 \times 10^{9}$/l	$4–15 \times 10^{9}$/l	1	$6–15 \times 10^{3}$/µl	$4–15 \times 10^{3}$/µl
Neutrophils (bands)	$0–0.3 \times 10^{9}$/l	$<0.3 \times 10^{9}$/l	1	$0–0.3 \times 10^{3}$/µl	$<0.3 \times 10^{3}$/µl
Neutrophils (seg)	$3–11.5 \times 10^{9}$/l	$2.5–12.5 \times 10^{9}$/l	1	$3–11.5 \times 10^{3}$/µl	$2.5–12.5 \times 10^{3}$/µl
Lymphocytes	$1.0–4.8 \times 10^{9}$/l	$1.5–7 \times 10^{9}$/l	1	$1.0–4.8 \times 10^{3}$/µl	$1.5–7 \times 10^{3}$/µl
Monocytes	$<1.3 \times 10^{9}$/l	$<0.85 \times 10^{9}$/l	1	$<1.3 \times 10^{3}$/µl	$<0.85 \times 10^{3}$/µl
Eosinophils	$<1.3 \times 10^{9}$/l	$<1.5 \times 10^{9}$/l	1	$<1.3 \times 10^{3}$/µl	$<1.5 \times 10^{3}$/µl
Basophils	Rare	Rare		Rare	Rare

Haemostatic values

	Dog	Cat
Prothrombin time (PT) (seconds)	7–12	7–12
Partial thromboplastin time (PTT) (seconds)	12–15	12–22

Urinalysis

	Dog	Cat
Specific gravity	1.001–1.070	1.001–1.080
pH	5.5–7.5	5.5–7.5
Sediment		
– leucocytes/hpf	0–5	0–5
– erythrocytes/hpf	0–5	0–5
– casts/hpf	0	0
Bilirubin	0–trace	0
Glucose/ketones	0	0
Protein (mg/dl)	<30	<20
Protein semiquantitative	0–trace/1+	0–trace/1+
Protein:creatinine ratio		
– normal	<0.2	<0.6
– questionable	0.2–1.0	0.6–1.0
– abnormal	>1.0	>1.0

Appendix (continued)

Serum chemistry

	SI Units (dog)	SI Units (cat)	Con. factor	Old Units (dog)	Old Units (cat)
ALT	7–50 u/l	7–50 u/l	—	7–50 u/l	7–50 u/l
Albumin	23–31 g/l	20–30 g/l	0.1	2.3–3.1 g/dl	2.0–3.0 g/dl
ALP	0–100 u/l	0–40 u/l	—	0–100 u/l	0–40 u/l
SIAP	<45 %			<45 %	
Amylase	400–2,000 u/l	400–1,650 u/l	—	400–2,000 u/l	400–1,650 u/l
Anion gap	8–19 mmol/l	9–21 mmol/l	—	8–19 mEq/l	9–21 mEq/l
Betahydroxybutyrate	<1 mmol/l	<1 mmol/l	—	n/a	n/a
Bile acids					
– fasting	<15 µmol/l	<15 µmol/l	0.41	<6.2 µg/ml	<6 µg/ml
– postprandial	<40 µmol/l	<40 µmol/l		<16 µg/ml	<16 µg/ml
Bilirubin - total	<6.8 µmol/l	0–2 µmol/l	0.059	<0.4 mg/dl	0–0.11 mg/dl
Calcium	2.2–2.7 mmol/l	2.1–2.6 mmol/l	4.0	8.8–10.8 mg/dl	8.4–10.4 mg/dl
Carbon dioxide - (TCO2)	17–27 mmol/l	13–25 mmol/l	1	17–27 mEq/l	13–25 mEq/l
Chloride	99–115 mmol/l	117–140 mmol/l	1	99–115 mEq/l	117–140 mEq/l
Cholesterol	3.2–6.5 mmol/l	1.9–3.9 mmol/l	38.8	124–252 mg/dl	74–151 mg/dl
Cobalamin (B12)	n/a	n/a	n/a	215–500 ng/l	200–1,680 ng/l
Cortisol					
– basal	25–260 nmol/l	15–200 nmol/l	0.036	0.9–9.4 µg/dl	0.54–7.2 µg/dl
– post-ACTH	200–660 nmol/l	130–450 nmol/l	0.036	7.2–24 µg/dl	4.7–16.3 µg/dl
Creatinine	20–110 µmol/l	40–120 µmol/l	0.0113	0.23–1.2 mg/dl	0.45–1.36 mg/dl
Folate	n/a	n/a	n/a	3.5–8.5 µg/l	13.4–38 µg/l
GGT	0–8 u/l	0–2 u/l	1	0–8 u/l	0–2 u/l
Globulin	27–40 g/l	26–51 g/l	0.1	2.7–4.0 g/dl	2.6–5.1 g/dl
Glucose	3.5–5.5 mmol/l	3.5–6.5 mmol/l	18	63–99 mg/dl	63–117 mg/dl
Lipase	0–300 u/l	0–250 u/l	1	0–300 u/l	0–250 u/l
Parathyroid hormone	2–13 pmol/l	0–4 pmol/l	n/a	n/a	n/a
Phosphate	0.8–2.0 mmol/l	1.1–2.3 mmol/l	3.1	2.5–6.2 mg/dl	3.4–7.1 mg/dl
Potassium	3.5–5.3 mmol/l	3.6–5.4 mmol/l	1	3.8–5.3 mEq/l	3.6–5.4 mEq/l
Sodium	140–153 mmol/l	145–156 mmol/l	1	140–153 mEq/l	145–153 mEq/l
Thyroxin (T4)	13–52 nmol/l	15–55 nmol/l	0.0777	1.0–4.0 µg/dl	1.2–4.3 µg/dl
TLI	n/a	n/a	n/a	5–35 µg/l	17–49 µg/l
Total protein	57–78 g/l	55–78 g/l	0.1	5.7–7.8 g/dl	5.5–7.8 g/dl
Triiodothyronine (T3)	0.7–2.3 nmol/l	0.14–1.25 nmol/l	64.9	45–149 ng/dl	9.1–81 ng/dl
Urea	3–7 mmol/l	3–9 mmol/l	2.8	8.4–19.6 mg/dl	8.4–25.2 mg/dl

NB: Cobalamin (B12), folate and TLI are always reported in Old Units, never in SI Units. Parathyroid hormone is always reported in SI units, never in Old Units.

Index

Index